D1789494

Jih-Yuan Chen
Susan L. Instone

Family Resilience and Functioning in Child with DMD

Jih-Yuan Chen
Susan L. Instone

Family Resilience and Functioning in Child with DMD

Functioning and Resilience in Families with Children with Duchenne Muscular Dystrophy

VDM Verlag Dr. Müller

Imprint

Bibliographic information by the German National Library: The German National Library lists this publication at the German National Bibliography; detailed bibliographic information is available on the Internet at http://dnb.d-nb.de.

Any brand names and product names mentioned in this book are subject to trademark, brand or patent protection and are trademarks or registered trademarks of their respective holders. The use of brand names, product names, common names, trade names, product descriptions etc. even without a particular marking in this works is in no way to be construed to mean that such names may be regarded as unrestricted in respect of trademark and brand protection legislation and could thus be used by anyone.

Cover image: www.purestockx.com

Publisher:
VDM Verlag Dr. Müller Aktiengesellschaft & Co. KG , Dudweiler Landstr. 125 a, 66123 Saarbrücken, Germany,
Phone +49 681 9100-698, Fax +49 681 9100-988,
Email: info@vdm-verlag.de

Zugl.: SanDiego, California, University of SanDiego, Diss., 2004

Produced in USA and UK by:
Lightning Source Inc., La Vergne, Tennessee, USA
Lightning Source UK Ltd., Milton Keynes, UK
BookSurge LLC, 5341 Dorchester Road, Suite 16, North Charleston, SC 29418, USA

ISBN: 978-3-639-06661-6

Contents

Introduction

Jih-Yuan Chen

Why do I interested in this special topic?

My interest in resilience started with the work on female adolescent offenders that I began at as a volunteer teacher in a respite institute. I found the score of resiliency scale in the group did not worse than the adolescent who were studying in the high school in my pilot study of adolescent resilience. I thought about that how the family structure or family system influenced the individuals' resilience. How did the adolescents and their families adapt to their diverse behavior? As mean time, I remembered in the interested study of Duchenne Muscular Dystrophy (DMD) eleven years ago, I had a chance to participate in a support group of families with child with Duchenne muscular dystrophy and have noted a considerable range of parent impact. When the work was being done in DMD, there were two types of DMD parents. There were "permissive" parents and "disrupted" parents. The difference between the two was striking. A different pattern of adaptation in the presence of uncommon stress, some of the parents decided to go outside to participate the self-group, but some of the parents could not go outside with their sons and became more distress.

Permissive parents have developed the association to organize the activities of the supporting group after I leaded them to support each other for eight times and searched for the relative finances to hold the multitude of the activities. Although the supporting group continued to develop, there were a few families broken but several families became more coherence and strengthen. The disrupted parents refused to pick up with the strangers, some of them isolated by themselves, a few of parents avoided their parental responsibilities or divorced, no any activity existed in the family. In the supporting group, there were several families who talked about how they adjusted the problems and adapted the progressive process when the child encountered the problems in the school or with their health. I think that resilience is manifest competence despite exposure to significant stressors.

My interests came from the following questions: What gave some DMD families the resilience to work through a crisis? Why were that some families fall apart when faced with adversities, while others thrived and became stronger? What were the qualities of these resilient families? And how did these families establish and maintain these strengths? I would like to explore above of those questions when I had participated the supporting group for the DMD child's family. Family is a complex social system. Numerous variables can be identified which explain family functioning.

I thought that resilience was one explanation for the difference in the two types of families. I used Chronic Impact and Coping Investment (CICI) to evaluate the impact of the parents, most parents' scored within the middle level of impact and coping strategies. The parents with higher impact or distress had a strong reaction to wish-fulfilling fantasy and information seeking. The concern and distress of these parents included: how to let child comfort and happy, exulting feeling, communicate with their couple and understand each other, keep close relationship with their couple, et al. The impact and coping strategies of the parent with DMD children, showed that the parent occurred concern and distress, needed help the other normal family children for their growth and development, emotion and behavior management, classes homework and make friend problem.

There was no significant difference between the impact of parents of children with DMD and parents of child with a fever. The fever group showed higher "stress," "conflict," and "help need". The DMD parents had a tendency to use wishfulling fantasy to cope. Impact was influenced by income and religion, and income and mother's age influenced coping strategies. Professional needs to manage the parents' conflict to provide information and resources, and to support the parents' emotional reactions to caring for a child with acute and chronic illness.

Why is important I need to study the specific area?

Having a chronic disease increases one's risk for secondary conditions (Adrian, 2002). A child with a disability means the child is deprived of physical and/or mental abilities. Disabling conditions are life-long and often require services from many agencies that increased financial costs, caregiver burden, social isolation, as well as restricting life –styles and career opportunities (Failla & Jones, 1991; Gottlieb, 1998).

The reciprocal impacts on the families are circular and continuous (Patterson, 2002). The sacrifices associated with chronic disease and disabilities are not temporary but become a way of life for the whole family with a disabled child. The family may have already depleted family energy and resources when the chronic condition deteriorates. The transition of a child with disabilities affects and is affected by the family social system. However, the slow and arduous illness course that can lead to parental strain has received little attention.

The philosophical and policy trends of de-institutionalization and normalization encourage families to raise children with developmental disabilities at home. Advances in medical science and changes in public policy have resulted in more disabled children supported in the community and at home. As more disabled children stay at home, families must become more diverse in their skills to meet the challenges and the special risks. In addition, the nation evolves into a multiracial, multicultural, and multilingual society.

Four important trends in a socio-historical context are: "diverse family forms," "changing gender roles and relations," "cultural diversity and socioeconomic disparity," and "varying and expanded family life cycle course" (Walsh, 1998, p.26). Despite transitions in their structure, families remain the most basic unit of society. There is encouraging evidence that research and resulting programs can contribute to the strength and resilience of all families.

More recently, attention has been focused on how a family copes with and adapts to a very difficult situation in an attempt to promote health and well being; to maintain the family's stability, social support, integration, and self-esteem; and to communicate with other families and medical teams. However, the slow and arduous illness course that can lead to parental strain or adaptation has received little attention in nursing.

Families involved with the extraordinary care taking demands of a disabled child are at risk for added stress, social isolation, and reduced feelings of autonomy. Researchers have observed that some individuals who experience a high degree of life stress remain healthy. They become actively involved in events, viewing them as meaningful. Life changes are viewed as opportunities for growth and development (Failla et al., 1991). This phenomenon can explain which resilience processes that adaptive families have developed to deal with their problems and cope effectively (Cohen, Slonim, Finzi, & Leichtentritt, 2002). However, a few articles in nursing applied the resilience model to evidence family adaptation of disabilities.

A change in one person has an effect on the whole family system. It is important for the professional to think systematically to use the resiliency model of family stress, adjustment, and adaptation to identify the risks and protective factors for the family with a disabled child. Family resilience is an important indication of overall adjustment and adaptation in the family with a disabled child. Exploring and developing the knowledge related to family resilience will help to develop and maintain the capacity of a family to be resilient, and will help to understand the influence of factors on family adaptation and resilience.

Part One

Getting Started: Selecting a Research Focus

Families of Children with Duchenne Muscular Dystrophy

Overview

Little is understood about how Taiwanese families' function when they have a child with Duchenne Muscular Dystrophy (DMD). Resilience, as well as hardiness, are important qualities found in families coping with other life stressors, and may also be factors in how DMD families function. The sacrifices families must make when a child has DMD - related disabilities are not temporary. Instead they become a way of life for the whole family and often require services from many agencies, which may result in increased financial costs, social isolation, as well as restriction of life-styles and career opportunities (Failla & Jones, 1991; Gottlieb, 1998; Patterson & McCubbin, 1983). The reciprocal impacts on the families are circular and continuous (Patterson, 2002).

Background and Significance

DMD, the second most common genetic disease in humans, is an X-linked disease of the muscle caused by mutation of the Xp21 gene. This gene encodes a rod like cytoskeletal protein called dystrophin that afflicts only boys who inherit the disease from their mothers (Emery, 1993; Nicholson, 1993). The world wide incidence, based on live male births, is around 200 to 300 x 10^{-6}, but the mutation rate is approximately 70 to 100 x 10^{-6} (Emery, 1993; Laing, 1993).

As children get older, DMD takes a slow and arduous course that leads to parental strains. The children's emotional responses in the form of problem behavior resulting from social isolation and poor interpersonal skills, has been found to predict maternal stress and anxiety (Huang & Dai, 1998; Nereo, Fee, & Hinton, 2003; Nereo & Hinton, 2003).

The progression of the children's disabilities induces the family to change and influences the entire family system (Botvin, Radford, & Neumann, 1984; Siegel, Davidson, Kornfeld, & McCready, 1983). Family structure, process, and functioning change the most as a result of the demands on family relationships, activities, and goals of the family social system (Thompson, Zeman, Fanurik, & Sirotkin-Roses, 1992). Families also change roles to meet the demands for achieving positive family functioning (Epstein, Bishop, Ryan, Miller, & Keitner, 1993). Some families adapt and others become depleted of family energy and resources; this difference has received little attention in the pediatric literature (Thompson et al., 1992).

The theoretical and empirical basis of a family-oriented approach has not been widely addressed, even in Taiwan, limiting the efforts of family health and human service providers involved in family health promotion. Health professionals have the responsibility to strengthen the family/child's coping resources and make the children's environment more accommodating to their special needs, as well as to assist their families to enrich their lives through interventions that enhance meaning and satisfaction in caregiving through positive experience and encounters.

The ability to maintain a balance between change and stability has been referred to as a measure of healthy family functioning. When families are able to utilize their strength and abilities, they are able to recover from the stress and challenge and minimize a negative outcome. The resilient family that adapts to stress has a higher level of functioning. Families that function well can solve problems, share affection, and meet the needs of individual family members.

If nursing professionals could evaluate family resilience and discuss interventions to support it, they could promote family functioning. And if the family of a DMD child can describe how they have dealt with the disability and anticipated loss, this might help others in similar situations to deal with their own sense of loss, fatigue, and distress. This study attempts to discover which family characteristics, supports, strengths, resources, and functioning buffer the impact of a stressful life and improve understanding of why some families thrives and other families do not. The findings of this study may contribute to the development of interventions that will help promote resilience in family members living with a child having DMD.

Little is understood about how families function when they have a child with DMD. Several studies focused on the impact and coping of families with disabled children. Given the research gaps, and lack of information about the functioning of culturally diverse families with a disabled child, this study involved a group of Taiwanese families to discover whether the factors associated with family functioning found in the literature were characteristic of them.

Literature Review

This literature focuses on Duchenne muscular dystrophy (DMD), Family stress in the child with chronic ill or handicapped, the impact of DMD on children's health, the impact of DMD on families, and cultural and religious meaning of DMD in Taiwan. With this foundation, the various conceptual models of family functioning will be examined and critiqued.

Duchenne Muscular Dystrophy

DMD is a neuromuscular disorder that presents as a chronic progressive disease that is physically incapacitating. It affects only boys and is inherited from their mothers (Emery, 1993). As carriers, women usually show no sign of the disease but they are capable of passing the condition on to their own sons. All affected daughters are carriers and the disease is never transmitted from father to son (Laing, 1993). In two thirds of cases there is a family history of the disorder; the remainder (70 to 100 x 10^{-6}) are spontaneous mutations (Emery, 1993; Laing, 1993). The genetic defect of DMD of the dystrophin (cDNA) is located in band XPp21 on the X chromosome (Francke et al, 1985). Absence of effective treatment for DMD has led to develop new approaches for carrier detection and prenatal diagnosis (Alcantara et al., 2001; Laing, 1993; Wang et al., 2001). Creatinine phosphokinase raised that is the best screen for neonatal diagnosis of DMD (Bradley, Parsons, & Clarke, 1993).

In Taiwan, the risk of a carrier having an affected child is one in four, with an incidence of 1 in 3000 to 1 in 3500 live male births; the mutation rate for DMD is about 1 in 10,000, which is very high in comparison with other genetic disorders (Laing, 1993). From 1981 to 2002, it is estimated that of 3,060,000 live male births there may have been approximately 1028 to 1199 DMD children born in Taiwan assuming each one lives to the age of 21 (Department of Health, 2001). The amount spent on medical care is over NT$ five million during the life of a DMD child (TMDA, 2002)

Even the muscles that control respiration and heartbeat fail, that leads to death, die before they reach 25 years of age (Koenig et al, 1987). The sacrifices are not temporary but become a way of life for the whole family. When chronic illness deteriorates into terminal illness, the family may have already depleted family energy and resources. However, the slow and arduous illness course that can lead to parental strains has received little attention. Chronic emotional stress experienced by families of DMD children was found to be a significant problem in the overall management of the illness (Buchanan, LaBarbera, Roelofs, & Olson, 1979). Doherty and Baptiste have stated that family functioning and interaction processes and patterns are crucial dimensions that have implications for enrichment theory and well practice (cited in Cole & Cole, 1993).

Family Stress in the Child with Chronic Ill or Handicapped

Patterson & McCubbin (1983) described that source of stress of families who have a chronically ill child included: 1). strained family relationship: over protectiveness, jeopardizing the child's development of independence; coalitions between the primary caretaker and the child; scapegoat and blaming of the child; overt or covert rejection of the child; worry about extended parenting/care taking responsibilities, sibling comparison and discrepancies; overall increase in intrafamily tension and conflict. 2). modifications in family activities and goals: reduced flexibility in the use of leisure time and restricted options for family vacations; less opportunity for both parents to pursue careers; worry and uncertainty about whether to have more children when the illness related to genetic factors. 3). the burden of increased tasks and time commitments: providing special diets, extra cleaning of equipment, providing daily therapy or treatment, extra appointments to medical facilities. 4). increased financial burden due to medical specialist consultations, hospitalizations, medications, equipment needs, therapy, with variety of insurance coverage affecting direct costs to families. 5). need for housing adaptation in terms of geographic proximity to adequate medical care. 6). social isolation: friends' and relatives' reaction; family embarrassment when there are visible abnormalities; limited mobility of the ill or handicapped child, unavailability of adequate child care, fear of accidents, exposure to infections or conditions; fear of accident, exposure to infections or conditions; limitations on social life. 7). medical concerns. 8). differences in school experiences. 9). grieving (Patterson et al., 1983, p. 25-26).

Most of parents their coping pattern for the chronic ill or handicaped child included: maintaining family integration, cooperation, and an optimistic definition of the situation; maintaining social support, self-esteem, and psychological stability; understanding the medical situation through communication with other parents and consultation with the medical staff (Patterson et al., 1983, p. 32).

The results showed that the stress model of the parents with DMD children, before touching the support group that included: (1) recognize the condition from health status change to realize the causes' factors that include unknown, surmise, rationalize, and acceptance of the mutation and sexual heredity, (2) help needs that include no barricade, social resource support (role substitute, coordinate, and long-term care), and medical information providing (causes and treatment, psychological adjustment, rehabilitative needs, and welfare system) and (3) overloads (physical, psychology, sleep disturbance, and powerlessness) (Chen & Jong, 2006).

Impact of DMD on Children's Health

Duchenne defined the disease as being characterized by progressive muscular weakness, first affecting the lower limbs and then later the upper limbs. The most obvious features in the early stage are enlargement of the calf muscle (called pseudohypertrophy) which is due to an excess of adipose and connective tissue, and a wadding gait (Emery, 1993). More often mothers notice that there is a delay in their child's learning to walk; in 56% of children with DMD walking was delayed until at least 18 months and roughly a quarter did not walk until they were at least 2 years old. In 90% of cases, the onset was before 5 years old. The affected child was never able to run properly (Emery, 1993). The major symptoms at onset were muscle weakness (31.8%) and falling down easily (31.8%). The onset of illness before age 5 was 36.4% (Chen, Chen, Jong, & Yang, 2002), and losing the ability to climb stairs occurred at a mean age of 9.3 +/- 1.4 years (range, 5.8 to 13.8 years) (Vignos, Wagner, Karlinchak, & Katirji, 1996).

The affected children experience progressive muscle weakness, manifested by difficulty getting from a sitting to a standing position. The first clinical symptoms such as waddling gait, walking unsteadily with a tendency to fall easily, walking on toes, difficulties of rising off the floor, squatting, and climbing stairs appear between 3 to 6 years of age (Hoffman, Brown, & Kunkel, 1987). In the early stage of the disease, this is evaluated by the Gower's maneuver, where the child tries to stand by using his hands to climb up his thighs, pushing down on them, and extending his hips and trunk in order to stand. An increase in interstitial connective tissue in the affected muscles, with the production of abundant fibrous and adipose issue, appears in the later stage (Emery, 1993).

General speaking, children are diagnosed with DMD between 3 and 11 years of age (Appleton & Nicolaides, 1995). The median age at diagnosis is 2 years (Siciliano et al., 1999). Most children are diagnosed with DMD after age two, but before their fifth birthday (Roland, 2000). Patients with DMD become unable to walk between 6 and 12 years, with a mean age of 10 years resulting in wheelchair dependency (Kilmer, Abresch, & Fowler, 1993). As the disease progresses and muscle weakness becomes more profound, the loss of hip extension and ankle dorsiflexion become the primary predictors of an inability to walk (Bakker, de

Groot, Beelen, & Lankhorst, 2002). Kyphoscoliosis develops and facial and neck muscles weaken. Eventually, he becomes confined to a wheelchair because of flexion contractures of the elbows, knees, and hips. By twelve, the feet may turn inward and downward (Emery, 2002).

Vignos et al. (1996) found that operative procedures combined with bracing and physical therapy, including daily passive stretching exercises and prescribed periods of standing and walking, were successful in controlling contractures of the lower extremities for as long as seven years after treatment. Their management allowed DMD boys to walk until a mean age of 13.6 years and to stand for an additional two years after the ability to walk with braces had been lost.

In addition, 20 % of the affected boys have an IQ of less than 70 (Emery, 2002). Thus, the disease affects the DMD child's physical strength, school achievement, and social activities with friends (Lue, Chen, Jong, & Lin, 1993). Most of the DMD children are lonely; they see other children enjoying friendships and an active social life, while their world is more restricted. The lack of physical activity and recreational opportunities can lead to the development of obesity as well as subsequent withdrawal, depression, and isolation (Adrian, 2002). Westernization of Taiwanese society has contributed to a rise in obesity as more people have access to high calorie fast food. In 1990, 25 % of boys and 18 % of girls in elementary school were obese (Lin, 1990). DMD children have a deficit of activities due to their weakened muscles; therefore, it is easier to become obese if they over eat. Their caregivers can exhaust their physical strength by taking care of their obese children.

The clinical definition of DMD includes becoming wheelchair bound by age 12, and death usually by the end of the third decade (Laing, 1993). The muscles that control respiration and cardiac function fail, leading to death. Respiratory failure invariably occurs in the second decade (Rideau et al., 1995). Death occurs by the early 20s or before they reach 25 years of age usually due to a simple cold or complicated pneumonia, and 9-50% die from cardiac failure (Emery, 1993; Parent Project Muscular Dystrophy, 2002). These children may require total care from their families for 6 to 8 years before they die. Survival to age 20 is estimated at 25% (Holroyd & Guthrie, 1986). Thus, the disease's progression has distressing consequences for the children and their families for 15-25 years (Firth, Gardner-Medwin, Hosking, & Wilkinson, 1983).

In a 40-year longitudinal study that evaluated the orthopedic treatment and physical therapy of 144 boys with DMD from 1953-1994, the major causes of death were pulmonary insufficiency (61%), pneumonia (31%), and cardiomyopathy (7%). Ninety-four percent of the patients had a functional classification of "confined to wheelchair" or "bed" at the time of death. The mean age at the time of death was 18.1 +/- 3.2 years (range, 11.8 to 24.6 years) during the 1960's, 19.0 +/- 2.8 years (range, 13.7 to 27.5 years) during the 1970's, and 18.8 +/- 3.4 years (range, 13.1 to 26.4 years) during the 1980's. Five of these subjects were between thirty-one and thirty-three years old and needed ventilator support (Vignos et al., 1996). Vignos et al (1996) reported "with the numbers available, we could not detect a significant difference among the treatment groups or time-periods with regard to the age at the time of death" (p .1849).

Anecdotal data over eight years from my clinical experience as a pediatric nurse in Taiwan confirms the progressive, debilitating nature of DMD. Most of these children are obese, lonely and living in worlds that are restricted, especially after they graduate from primary school and do not attend high school. Practical problems such as transportation, difficulty with the physical labor of lifting, the need for increased medical attention, and the tremendous financial burden upon the family have all been observed to some degree. How these burdens affect Taiwanese families' ability to function, however, are not well understood.

Impact of DMD on the Family

Family Perception of Having a DMD Child

Some studies have indicated that parents are significantly concerned about problems relating to the care of DMD children including the practical problems of daily living, emotional problems, the drain on other personal relationships, and the exclusion of other family needs (Firth et al., 1983; Siegel et al., 1983).

About 62% of the parents (N = 65) in one study experienced these problems: lifting, housing, difficultly using public transportation, and concern about what they should tell their sons about the disease (Firth et al., 1983). In another study, the major needs of 61 parents with a DMD child in Taiwan were getting information (71%) about coping with the disease, accessing health care (68%), the progression of disease (65%); and support groups (48%). The major concerns were how to comfort the child and help him be happy (89%), how to maintain a close couple relationship (79%), and how to overcome exhaustion (73%) (Chen, Chen, Jong, Yang, & Lue, 2003).

Some parents are able to accept and adapt to the disability by finding a meaningful pattern of life. Gagliardi (1991) found that the response of families living with a DMD child were characterized by various stages of adaptation. The "recognition stage" lead to "disillusionment" and the realization that "society confirms the impossibility of normalcy". Families then moved to the "work out stage" to adjust to the disability and maintain the "dynamic of the family: who's disabled anyway", to by adjusting to "a smaller world", and then deciding whether to "let go or hang on", with the realization that "things must change" (pp.162-163). The intervention implications of these studies include restructuring psychosocial services for the entire family and providing a network of liaison services to assist the family as the disease progresses.

Family Stress and Family Coping

The prior studies indicated that over half of the families had psychological adjustment problems (Buchanan, LaBarbera, Roelofs, & Olson, 1979; Thompson et al., 1992) because of the stressors of their sons' decreasing independent abilities and behavior problems (loneliness and depression), marital conflict, increase in daily chores, duties, and responsibilities of caring for the child, and lack of support from extended family and school personnel. These problems lead the parents to utilize denial, isolation, magical thinking, or overprotection and to feel a sense of guilt and hopelessness. A study of 112 mothers found that their stress was elevated because of negative behaviors of their DMD children, especially in social interactions (Nereo et al., 2003). On the other hand, 75 % of families reported a positive couple relationship and 72 % of parents with DMD children were satisfied with their marital status (Chen et al., 2002).

The chronic stress of living with a child who has a progressively deteriorating illness often motivates families to seek emotional support from groups and institutions around them. Extended families and schools are the major support systems. But some of the grandparents may blame the disability on in-laws, or the mothers may blame themselves for carrying the defective genes. Arguments focused on how to care for the child, discipline, constant fatigue from the labor involved, and interference from the extended family have been described (Buchanan et al., 1979).

In addition, the children often were placed in special education classes to avoid obvious physical competition with normal boys and to allay parents' fear that their children were being abused in public schools. Some of the parents also believed that some teachers did not understand their children and tended to spoil them, refusing to discipline them and excusing their behavior because of the illness, or expecting more from them than they could physically perform. On the other hand, the use of homebound teachers for these boys contributed to their social isolation (Buchanan et al., 1979).

Parental coping by preserving their own emotional well-being, reducing family conflict, and improving family supportiveness showed a significant positive correlation with a measure of parent adjustment (Buchanan et al., 1979). Parents with higher monthly incomes who lived in cities were both more aggressive and more afraid of other's criticism. The children's ability to cope was compromised because they were isolated, could not get peer support, and could not freely express their thought and feelings and easily felt rejected (Chen et al., 2003). Another study found that parents with disabled children revealed significantly more avoidant coping, lower sense of coherence, and less emphasis on family members' interrelations and personal growth than did the control group (Margalit, Raviv, & Ankonina, 1992).

Reaction of Siblings

Siblings may need to change their role to care for their affected brothers. Botvin et al. (1984) found that there may be a tendency for older sisters to adopt a maternal role and to overprotect their ill brother. In their study, sisters tended to be very defensive in response to the actions and attitudes of people outside the family toward their sibling. Siblings may experience some degree of emotional distress and they may need help with feelings of jealousy because the affected child seems to get more attention (Botvin et al., 1984). However, Nereo et al. (2003) reported that stress of DMD children was not significantly different from that of their siblings.

Disclosure Issues

Fitzpatrick and Barry (1986) found that most parents were unable to discuss the condition with their sons. None of the boys had asked about the progression of their disorder. Some siblings were informed of the affected boy's condition but they were not told about the disease progression. Fitzpatrick et al. (1990) conducted a retrospective case-control study to compare the patterns of communication and use of professional support systems in Irish and

American families with DMD boys. The results indicated that difficulty in communication with their spouse (73% Irish and 24% American) and with their affected sons (94% Irish and 52% American) were reported by significantly more Irish parents than by their American counterparts. More Irish parents (56%) never talked about DMD with their sons.

Informational Needs of Families

Smith, William, Sibert, and Harper (1990) found that only 68% of the mothers (N=201) in their study were aware that infants could be screened during the neonatal period, and more multiparous than primparous mothers were aware of such screening. Ninety-four percent of these mothers would accept a screening test for DMD, and 75 % would want to know soon after birth whether their babies had a disabling condition. Seventy percent of these mothers would consider termination of their pregnancy for medical reasons. In fact, DNA studies of cultured amniotic fluid cells at 14 weeks gestation, the absence of the X-chromosomal fragment of DXYS19X located in XY21.2-pter or Xp22.3 and analysis of several STR loci of dystrophin, followed by multiplex PCR, lead to the diagnosis of a male fetus affected by DMD; and quantitative multiplex PCR confirmed the deletion in female carriers (Jakubiczka et al., 2000). In addition, Chen et al. (2003) found that families also needed information about physiotherapy, genetic issues, and support groups to prevent them from selecting useless rituals or remedies for their DMD children.

Summary. These studies suggest that emotional support, parent education, and other services can improve satisfaction and communication to help families resolve their problems and function better. The data also suggest that little effort has been made to inform parents about neonatal screening so that early diagnosis and supportive care are not delayed unnecessarily.

Cultural and Religious Meaning of DMD in Taiwan

Common Cultural and Family Value

By 1970, Taiwan had undergone a transformation from an agricultural society to an industrial and technological country. Many Taiwanese families have become smaller nuclear families while maintaining traditional Chinese spiritual beliefs. These include life philosophies of "giving birth to new life (生生不息 Sheng-sheng buo-hsin)", "unity of heaven and man (天人合一 T'ien- Jem houi-yii)", "way of heaven (天道 T'ien-tao)", and "way of man (人道 Jem-tao)". This spiritual foundation gives meaning to the lives of Taiwanese families as they are "playing out one's inherent nature" (盡性 chin-hsing) (*Traditional Chinese Culture in Taiwan: Philosophy*, 2002, para 4). These beliefs may help parents understand the meaning of their child's illness and help them function by developing hardiness to overcome their gradual loss.

In Chinese societies the son carries the family lineage. There are three things that are unfilial and having no progeny is the greatest of these. Chinese lineage reflects and reinforces structural features of Chinese society and functions to maintain that society (Freedman, 1979). Therefore, having a disabled son who will die prematurely is a severe blow to Taiwanese families.

The values of dragon son / phoenix daughter. According to an idiom of Mandarin "wang nan tso lung, wang nu tso huang," one "hopes their son will become a dragon, and hopes their daughter will become a phoenix." "Dragon in this context means success for the male in any endeavor; phoenix for the female means she will get a good education, have a good career, and marry a successful man" (Marsh, 1996, p. 284). Parents' attitudes about socializing their children are defined by their ideas about discipline and corporal punishment as a means of bringing children up properly for a successful life. According to Marsh (1996), two thirds of parents believed that their children needed more discipline and thought that in order to bring children up to be fine human beings, physical punishment was sometimes necessary. For families with children with DMD, how to deal with emotional problems without using physical punishment becomes an important challenge.

The values of harmony and yin-yang. Harmony, including the concepts of yin and yang and the five basic forces (metal, wood, water, fire, and earth), are important for understanding health and illness in Chinese culture. These concepts imply that human beings and nature are interrelated and interdependent to maintain harmony. To re-establish the harmonious state, traditional Chinese medicine uses herbs and food to correct the disturbance and imbalance in the body systems. People in Taiwan prefer to receive western medicine for treating acute illnesses, but in the recovery stage, they prefer to use traditional Chinese medicine to restore energy and balance in their bodies. The parents of children with DMD also wish to find harmonious therapies for their children.

Buddhism

According to the Buddhist philosophy of life, life is pain and suffering because of ignorance and desires. Disability is a consequence of deeds done in previous lives and is associated with evil spirits or karma. Therefore, when a son has a disability and suffers an early death, both the child and the family have to tolerate the pain and discomforts and undergo treatment together. For example, family members go to the temple to get a special charm as a blessing from Buddha to keep away evil spirits, to experience pain or pleasure, and to deal with the positive and/or negative reactions to the child's disability. Most Taiwanese mothers make the sacrifice required to care for their sons if they are sustained by their religion, folk beliefs, or social support. An added burden for them is the cultural expectation that they will also care for their husband's aging parents.

Changing Demographics in Taiwan

Economic Impact and National Health System

Taiwan's ratio of economically active people to the retired has begun to fall, imposing an increasing by onerous burden on the younger working population (Gold, 1996). Since the global economy has declined, a young couple might have difficultly buying a house if they have no support. These financial burden are even more challenging for families with DMD children (Bothwell et al., 2002) although national health insurance covers all residents in Taiwan.

Recently, the government and private organizations have developed daycare centers for working mothers. In addition, there are respite services for DMD children, except in rural areas, but these still need to be better organized. National health insurance has reimbursed home nursing services since 1996. As a result, in-home nursing services have become a rapidly growing health industry. The number of home nursing agencies increased from 27 in 1993 to 125 in 1997 (Long-Term Care Profession Association of ROC, 1997).

Urbanization

Highly urbanized, often freakishly ugly high-rise apartment blocks and factories are crammed together. There has been little advance in macro-level planning or co-ordination, posing tremendous problems of utilities, service and green spaces. As a developing society, Taiwan has seen continuous and rapid rural out-migration that tended to rely on and maintain ties with kin in the cities (Greenhalgh, 1984). While an excellent transportation and telecommunications infrastructure has been created for able-bodied persons, public access for the disabled has not been created developed, keeping DMD children and their families socially isolated.

Education System

Revolutionary changes in the educational system in Taiwan have made it possible for most people (over 70 %) to enter higher education after senior high school. However, most DMD children have had to drop out of school when parents cannot provide transportation, children cannot pass the entrance examination, or the children's health is poor. It is not enough to supply one-on-one teaching at home for the DMD children, although some cities in Taiwan have systems to teach at home. The quality of life of the children and their families has to be considered when DMD children are permanently absent from the school.

Summary

In summary, Taiwanese families utilize spiritual beliefs, especially those from Buddhism, to explain their child's disability and cope with the loss of a successful son. In addition, these children and their families remain isolated because of a lack of information, transportation, and support services. Despite these concerns, some families have maintained positive relationships in the family. In order to better understand what else these families need to function better, several models of family functioning will be explored.

Family Society in Taiwan

Disabling conditions are life-long, and often require services from many agencies, and they increase financial costs, caregiver burden, and social isolation, as well as restricting life-styles and career opportunities (Failla & Jones, 1991; Gottlieb, 1998; Patterson & McCubbin, 1983). The reciprocal impacts on the families are circular and continuous (Patterson, 2002). The sacrifices associated with chronic disease and disabilities are not temporary but become a way of life for the whole family with a disabled child. The family may have already depleted family energy and resources when the chronic condition deteriorates. The transition of a child with disabilities affects and is affected by the family social system.

A family in Taiwan is patrilineal, patriarchal, and virilocal (Jordan, 1972). The lives of families in Taiwan are expected to follow the traditional Chinese cultural thought. It is necessary to understand how Chinese philosophical thought and modern cultural exchange influence the social system and women's roles. These changes in contemporary Taiwan and will affect future family life: "diverse family forms," "changing gender roles and relations," "cultural diversity and socioeconomic disparity," and "varying and expanded family life cycle course" (Walsh, 1998, p.26). This paper will explore the geography and the history of Taiwan, discuss Chinese philosophical views, and discuss the cultural and social systems that affect family life.

Geography and History of Taiwan

Geography of Taiwan

Taiwan is a mountainous island, situated in the Pacific Ocean about 160 kilometers from the southeastern coast of mainland China, which is located as a regional commercial hub. There are 87 small islands, such as Quemoy, Matsu and Pescadors, scattered around Taiwan in the Pacific Ocean (*Geography*, 2002b). The total area of the province is about 36,000 square kilometers. Shaped like tobacco leaf, the main island of Taiwan is 394 kilometers in length and 144 kilometers wide at its broadest point (*Taiwan geography*, 2002). High mountains and hills are centered in the east and central part of the island. The plains are almost all in the west part of Taiwan. High temperature, large amount of rain and wind are the climate features of Taiwan. The annual average temperature is about 72 degrees. During the summer and autumn there are typhoons, which bring heavy rain and often cause a lot of damage (Teta, 1971).

History of Taiwan

Taiwan was first incorporated into the Chinese empire in 1206 under the Yuan dynasty as a protectorate. In 1684 it was added to the coastal province of Fujian-by which time a number of other powers were also staking their claim. The Portuguese gave Taiwan the name Formosa that declared the island "beautiful island." The Spanish and the Dutch had occupied Taiwan for a brief time (1624-1653). In 1653 to 1661 Ming Dynasty took over and Koxinga (Cheng, Cheng-Kung) defeated the Dutch and landed at Tainan, Anping in 1661. In 1684 to 1780 Taiwan became an island frontier of the Ching dynasty. Until 1895, the Japanese were the new colonial masters of Taiwan for 50 years after the War between China and Japan, when China ceded control to Japan, making an indelible mark on Taiwan. After War II, the Nationalist Chinese Government reclaimed Taiwan (*Taiwan introduction 2000*, 2000). After December 1949, mainland China fell into the hands of Communists. The National government of the Republic of China moved to Taiwan, and became populated with immigrants from Fujian and Guangdung provinces on China's southeastern coast. The ethnic group includes: Taiwanese 84%, Chinese 14%, and aborigine 2% (Taiwan Geography, 2001). Mandarin is the official language of Taiwan.

Traditional Chinese Culture in Taiwan

Chinese Philosophical Thought: Creative Life Force in the Universe and Human Society

The major famous philosophical thoughts of ancient China are "Confucian, Taoist, Mohist, Dialectician, and Legalist School of Thought." Confucianism, Buddhism, and Neoconfucianism have influenced China's neighbors, including Japan, Korea, and Vietnam (*Traditional Chinese culture in Taiwan: Philosophy*, 2002). The great emphasis of China's philosophers are "Way of Heaven" (天道 Tien-tao) and the "Way of Man" (人道 Jem-tao). The concept of "heaven" and "man" are new life and new values that are constantly brought forth in the universe and in human society. The former is indicated as "birth of new life" (生生 sheng-sheng), and the latter as "playing out one's inherent nature" (盡性 chin-hsing) (*Traditional Chinese culture in Taiwan: Philosophy*, 2002).

The life philosophies of "giving birth to new life" and "unity of heaven and man" lead the Chinese, on the one hand, to stress ethical feelings such as "benevolence: love for all"

(仁 jen)," ``courtesy'' or ``ceremony (禮 li): requires rational forethought and self-restraint (*Traditional Chinese culture in Taiwan: Philosophy*, 2002). Benevolence", and "Courtesy" or "Ceremony" are inherent in man's nature, and bring forth such virtues as filial respect for one's parents and fraternal duty toward one's siblings (孝悌 hsiao ti), loyalty and empathy for others (忠恕 chung shu), and acting in good faith (信義 hsin I) (*Traditional Chinese culture in Taiwan: Philosophy*, 2002).

Only through filial love and care of one's parents, and loving kindness to one's children is one better able to extend one's experience of living from the past to the present and into the future, forming an unbroken stream of life and expressing the creative continuity of the universe (*Traditional Chinese culture in Taiwan: Philosophy*, 2002).

Religions of Taiwan

Buddhism, Taoism, folk belief and superstition form the broad base of Taiwanese religious culture. Most Chinese go to temple to pray for peace; over 90 percent of Taiwan's residents are either self-described animists, Buddhists, or Taoists (Chu & Wen, 1975). Most families perform the filial duties of ancestral worship. Chinese folk religion emphasizes stability and harmony rather than change and emphasizes the importance of order in interpersonal relations in the real world (Chu, 1992).

Several families attempted to improve their financial fortunes and the health of their family members by means of a rite called a Shietuu; the term means "thanking the earth" but with correcting family misfortunes through exorcism; or performed a rite that is known as "changing luck", which was done in the public temple (Jordan, 1972). On important occasions, such as when a son or daughter takes the university entrances examination, people visit temples to present petitions and solicit divine assistance. Generally, the major reasons why Taiwan's families attend temple is for information about fertility, gestation and birth, growth of adolescence, adulthood responsibilities, seniority and old age, death and the ritual process of funerals, life after death (Habito, 2002). In general, people offered food and wine and burned paper money to the Gods, to the ancestors, or to wandering ghosts at special occasions (Jordan, 1972).

There are also many Christians (4.5%) (including Catholic and Protestant: 2.5%) inhabitants on the island (*Taiwan geography*, 2001). Christianity has a major impact on the cultural values and social relations. Families in Taiwan not only greatly value harmonious and stable family relations, but also they take Chinese-style family relations to be a kind of ideal (Chu, 1992).

Chinese Patterns of Ritual. The characteristic Chinese approach to the world of humans, gods, and things, has its roots in the Chinese family and kinship system. Festivals on the birthdays of the local gods are the important structuring element of local life. The different religious specialists perform rituals during the occasions. The Ritual Masters and the spirit mediums work in the courtyard that is an important place of sacrifice. People set animals, vegetables, and fruit substances out in this space. Taoist or Buddhist priests in the temples serve a great number of individuals over a wide area and perform elaborate classical rituals.

In face of continuing government restrictions and prohibitions, religious activities in city are extremely limited by government supervision and rapidly changing social customs. The ritual procession, the offerings, and the theatre are individually interrelated. There is a rhythm and a flow of intensities throughout the course of the entire community performance. Each community brings its own desires to bear upon the selection of elements from the regional culture and ritual tradition (Dean, 1993). They changed the ritual to fit into their new society, even creating new gods and rituals to meet their needs for security and survival.

Traditional Chinese Values Filial Piety (Xiao Tao)

The tradition of filial piety and reverence for age are basic norms underlying Chinese family organization. Families play a major role in providing older people with informal care and support. "The idealized form of filial piety in Chinese tradition implies deep loyalty, respect, and devotion by children to parents"(Ng, Phillips, & Lee, 2002). In Chinese societies the son carries the family lineage. There are three things that are unfilial and having no progeny is the greatest of these. Chinese lineage reflects and reinforces structural features of Chinese society and functions to maintain that society (Freedman, 1979).

Meal rotation involves married sons taking turns according to a fixed schedule in the provision of meals for their parents. In other words, it is means whereby parents are supported by their adult male heirs. Equal sharing of the responsibility of supporting parents by sons is a Chinese cultural concept. The Chinese consider supporting parents to be a natural, unalterable principle of life (Hsieh, 1992).

Social System in Taiwan

Demographic Change in Taiwan's Society

Over the past four decades, the demographics, standard of living, occupational structure, stratification system, life style, and gender relations have undergone fundamental changes. Annual population growth (0.80 %) and life expectancy rates (76 years, male: 73 years, female: 79 years) put Taiwan between the World Bank's "upper-middle" and "high income" economies. The natural rate of population increase has fallen below one percent, with the total fertility rate falling (Gold, 1996 in China Quartely; *Taiwan geography*, 2001).

The high savings rate helped families deal with the absence of any kind of universal medical care or social security program for the elderly (Gold, 1996). Taiwan's ratio of economically active people to the retired has begun to fall, imposing an increasing onerous burden on the younger working population (Gold, 1996).

The cause of death has changed, reflecting people succumbing to lengthy illnesses requiring expensive care. The government passed a politically controversial National Health Insurance Law effective from 1 March 1995. It calls for mandatory participation and covers everyone. The employer must pay 60 percent of the insurance premium, employees pay 30 percent, and the government pays 10 percent (Chan & Yang, 1995; Liu, 1995).

Based on quality of life indicators, Taiwan ranks among the world's most developed societies. Not only has calorie consumption risen, but also fat consumption has increased (*Directorate- General of Budget, Accounting and Statistics*, 1993). The growing food industry in Taiwan is one sign of its development. As more people have access to high calorie fast food, fat consumption has increased. There were 25 % of boys and 18 % of girls in elementary school were obese (Lin, 1990). As a result of fat consumption, environmental pollution and stress, diseases such as cancer, cerebral vascular, and heart disease are increasing (*Cause of death statistics*, 2001).

In addition, accident and suicide events are increasing and the death rate by this cause is higher than other countries in Taiwan. So health professionals must to emphasize that people maintain balance by relaxing programs, remind people to comply with the rules of transportation, and behavior control. Social support and relationship network might help people to share their feelings and avoid being alone by separation.

Geographical Changes in Taiwan

Highly urbanized, often freakishly ugly high-rise apartment blocks and factories are crammed together. There have been little advance macro-level planning or co ordination, posing tremendous problems of utilities, service and green spaces. Widely speculative rise in land prices spawned a fury of new building, with condominium buyers putting their money down before construction began, and the investors using this cash to start up new ventures (Gold, 1996). Since the global economy has declined, a young couple might have difficultly buying a house if they have no support. This had lead to new buildings becoming vacant after 2000. Vacant buildings may make problems in public security.

Urbanization in Taiwan

As a developing society, Taiwan has seen continuous and rapid rural out-migration that tended to rely on and maintain ties with kin in the cities (Greenhalgh, 1984). Excellent transportation and telecommunications infrastructure have avoided the severe gaps, so during periods of economic hardship many rural migrants returned to the countryside until things improved (Gold, 1996). The development of the rural area has slowed and the diversity between rural and urban has increased. Health problems may become different and demands of health care system may have to be reevaluated.

Education in Taiwan

Education in Taiwan has changed since the early periods of the Republic. Children below age six may attend kindergarten or nursery schools. Recently, the government and private organizations have developed daycare centers for working mothers. The elementary schools are free and include nine grades. Past three decades, students take examinations to determine whether they will go to an academic high school, a three-year vocational high school, a five-year junior college, a five-year normal college to prepare for a teaching college at an elementary school; or they will end his or her education and find employment in industry or agriculture. A student who does poorly on the high school entrance exam may retake the exam after tutorial work or may enter a private high school. Only those students with highest scores (10%) gain admission to the university. Yet only 35% (1971-1975) graduate in the four-or five-year period (Smith, 1977-1979).

Students spend two or three hours per day in study beyond the six hours spent in the classroom. Also numerous communities have private tutors. These study centers meet from 7 to 10 p.m. daily and the senior high school students engage in private moonlighting pedagogical quizzes on their lessons. Once a year, the entrance examination is opened to all. It is competitive and fairly graded. One's wealth, family background, or prior education does not affect the score. There is no indication of favoritism or dishonesty in this process

Revolutionary changes in the educational system in Taiwan have made it possible for most people (over 70 %) to enter higher education after senior high school. Almost all vocational schools and 5-year normal colleges have become 4-year colleges or universities or combined with a 2-year technical college. All will transform completely in a couple of years. The students are also able to apply for entrance into higher education. There are more scholars seriously studying in Taiwan as the quality of faculty increases. The ultimate goal of any educational system is to bring about self-actualization to the individual and harmony to the society. Promoting the level of education will induce people to compete in occupations that may let more people feel stress and influence the harmony of the family.

Family Life in Contemporary Taiwan

Family Structure Change in Taiwan

Taiwan's family structure and behavior have changed consistent with sociological predictions about the relationship between industrialization and family structure. Nuclear families early on replaced stem and extended families as the most common patterns, and many couples are opting not to have children (Thornton & Lin, 1994; Yuan, 1993). Since 1984, the birth rate has fallen below the replacement level, prompting the government in May 1995 to urge people to marry earlier and raise the birth rate back to two children per couple (Cheng, 1995; Lin, 1995). Family network might be an important factor in reproductive behavior in societies undergoing rapid social and economic change (Chuang, 1992). The government in Taiwan found that the birth rate decreased, aged people increased and the life expectancy prolonged, so the government has tried to make policies that encourage fertility (*Making policy to encourage fertility*, 2002).

With schooling and increased employment opportunities, young people are spending more time outside the home, and also residing elsewhere, both before or after marriage (Thornton, Chang, & Sun, 1984). More households have both husband and wife working, although women continue to bear a double burden of having most of the responsibility for housework and child care as well as doing a job outside the home (Farris, 1993). 70 % of college-educated married women work outside the home. Professional women attempted to juggle complicated careers while trying to meet society's expectations of remaining simple, in the process reinforcing the existing social ideology and power relations between genders (Cambridge, 1995). Even with today's rapid educational modernization and economic growth and the trend toward female employment outside of home, traditional inter-generational lineal relations are still maintained (Chang, Freedman, & Sun, 1981).

Preschools have emerged in recent years as an alternative means of assisting working couples with small children. The government has promoted a sexual equality in the Work Place Act, which includes provisions on maternity and paternity leave (Chiu, 1996; Yun, 1993). Although Taiwan's extended family has declined, Taiwanese maintain ties with their larger family network. They viewed these obligations more as voluntary actions than moral responsibilities, and improved transport, communication, affluence and leisure time, plus a desire to return to their roots and state emphasis on traditional family values are possible reasons explaining increased contact, in particular for events such as weddings, Chinese New Year, and ancestor worship (Marsh & Hsu, 1994).

The middle class has now sparked a strong emphasis on leisure-time activities. Besides shopping and elaborate meals, time-consuming pastimes such as golf and karaoke also enjoy great popularity. The modernization of transport has facilitated travel around the island (Gold, 1996). As result, the families need other health care agencies to take care of the chronically ill or disabled members, women with newborns within the first month in Taiwan, or the terminal ill members. Caregiver training programs become important strategies for the modern family. In addition, to know how traditional family structures and family values have changed during the process of modernization in Taiwan, it is important to look at changing family structure, persistence and changes of family values, intergenerational relationship, and elder care (Shih, 2002).

Social Structure and Social Change

Industrialization and urbanization have brought many social changes in business; industry, population, and education have a great impact on family structure and family values in Taiwan in recent decades. In the process of social transformation, many Taiwanese families are slowly adapting to a nuclear family form. However, the majority of the elderly still reside with their children. The number of elderly persons under day care had increased by 96.6%; and the number of elderly persons under home care had increased from 161,000 persons to 621,000. The safety networks for the elderly will be more comprehensive in the coming future (Social Welfare). To encourage families to take care of their disabled elderly members, National Health Insurance has reimbursed home nursing services since 1996. As a result, in-home nursing services have become a rapidly growing health industry. The number of home nursing agencies increased from 27 in 1993 to 125 in 1997 (Long-Term Care Profession Association of ROC, 1997).

Career Development and Family Organizations

Because of rapid economic development, there has been a significant growth of women's labor force participation, which is strongly associated with division of labor and decision making power within the family. It is worth noting how the changing family organization and social changes affect family members' career development, kinship system, and marriage formation and dissolution, as well as the changing working pattern among married women, changing marriage patterns, family and kinship system, and changing gender structure in the family (Shih, 2002).

Dynamics of Marriage Change

Betrothal was the first step in the marriage that established the bonds of affinity between the two families. A series of gift exchanges began with betrothal. Reciprocal gift giving creates social relations of solidarity between social equals. When one of the givers gives more than the other, their relations become asymmetrical with the givers of the greater gifts left in the better position. The patrilocal grand form of marriage in traditional Chinese society dramatized an ideal situation in which the family of the bride would have given the greater gifts. The gift of the bride herself and her dowry would bring the bride's family up to a level of approximate social equality with the family of the groom (Whyte, 1992).

In addition, the pattern of change in the process of mate choice shifts from arranged marriages to love matches. The women have played a major role in the decision to marry, meet their husband directly or through an introduction from peers, rather than parents, to have a date prior to marriage, to have one or more romances, and to recall feeling in love prior to marriage. Introductions and parental influence still played some role (Whyte, 1992). Although the role of parents in controlling mate choice has decreased, they still exercise considerable influence over marriage and even dating, although in consultation with children.

Many women rarely or never have dated their husbands prior to marriage, and most women did not have other serious boyfriends or marriage prospects besides the men they eventually married in the earlier stage. During 1950s, further dramatic shifts toward greater freedom of mate choice occurred in the lives of women who married. Through Western films and television shows, contact with foreign teachers, travel abroad, and in other ways, Chinese are being exposed to alternative models of behavior involving much greater youth autonomy, causal dating and premarital intimacy (Whyte, 1992).

Life Cycle of Women

A woman left her family on marriage and contributed children to the group into which she married. Her domestic services, her fertility, and her chief ritual attachments were transferred from one family to another (Freedman, 1958). Based on field interview done by Wolf and his wife research into the life of Taiwanese countrywomen in the past decades showed the following results:

In the past 5 decades, the adoption of girls (sim-pua means little daughters-in-law) was a common way of obtaining a bride for a son and a dutiful daughter-in-law for a family. Quiet wealthy families adopted infants to raise as wives for their sons because they felt that incorporating a female from outside the family was less disruptive if it was accomplished when she was still a baby and could be raised to be a dutiful wife (Wolf, 1972).

In addition, in old Chinese society it is common for widows to remain faithful to their deceased husbands, never remarrying. It is not easy to find a man who is willing to marry into a woman's family, although few men are required to change their surnames to that of their wives and to abandon their own ancestors; a man who has married into his wife's family is accused of doing just that (Wolf, 1972).

A woman must provide the links in the male chain of descent, but she will never appear in anyone's genealogy as that all-important name connecting the past to the future. If she died before she is married, her tablet will not appear on her father's altar; although she was a temporary member of his household, she was not a member of his family. A man is born into his family and remains a member of it throughout his life and even after his death (Wolf, 1972).

When a young woman marries, her formal ties with the household of her father are severed. Her father or brother throw water to indicate that she, like the water, may never return. If she is ill treated by her husband's family, her father's family may deal with it, but unless her parents are willing to bring her home and support her for the rest of the life, there is little they can do beyond shaming the other family (Wolf, 1972).

As long as her mother is alive, the daughter will continue her contacts with her father's household by as many visits as her new situation allows. No matter where she lives she must at least be allowed to return at New Year. After her mother dies her visits become perfunctory. Her brother plays an important ritual role throughout her life. She may gradually lose contact with her sisters as she and they become more involved with their own children, but her relations with her brother continue. As when she dies, the coffin cannot be closed until her brother determines to his own satisfaction that she died a natural death and her husband's family did everything possible to prevent it (Wolf, 1972).

Family Size

In the past two decades, Taiwan parents have changed the way they raised their children. As family size decreases, Taiwanese parents are anxious to provide their children with enrichment opportunities, such as music, art, travel, and sports. As a result, they send their children to after school programs. In addition, parents focus on the skills their children's need to pass the entrance exam for admission into higher education. However, the Taiwanese families have changed in other ways.

Whereas in the past, the family valued filial piety, now families are shifting their attention to the children; as a result, the nuclear family has more time together so the relationship between parents and children becomes the strongest. While some of the changes are beneficial the structure of Taiwanese society must change to accommodate elder care and children care.

Opportunity for Women

Females typically work before marriage and withdraw from the job market at marriage or at childbirth. Later a substantial proportion may re-enter the labor force after child-rearing stage which results in a twin peak labor force participation trend for females (Yi & Chien, 2002).

Hopeful Future

In the past two decades, Taiwan parents have changed the way they raise their children. According to an idiom of Mandarin "wang nan tso lung, wang nu tso huang," this means that "hope their son will become a dragon, and hope their daughter will become a phoenix". Dragon in this context means success for the male in any endeavor; phoenix for the female means she will get a good education, have a good career, and marry a successful man (Marsh, 1996).

Parents' attitudes about socializing their children are particular to their ideas about discipline and corporal punishment as a means of bringing children up properly for a successful life. Two thirds of parents believed that their children needed more discipline and thought that in order to bring up children up to be fine human beings, physical punishment is sometimes necessary (Marsh, 1996).

Ministry of Education reiterated that punishment is forbidden in school. Teacher should correct the students with patience and love instead of physical punishment. Although physical punishment is not allowable under the government, it actually exists (Chen, 1991). Marsh (1996) found that the "factors increased the log odds of favoring corporal punishment for children including more education, being younger and more likely to be involved in bringing up children at the present time, having a history of occupational immobility or downward mobility, and having relatively low income (p.290)."

Current Trends and Future Dimensions

Taiwan's society today is dependent on modern technology, and enjoys a modern life style, freedom and civil liberties and a political democracy (Mayer, 1996). It has evolved increasingly to resemble that of other industrialized nations: urban, mobile, structurally complex education, consumerist, plugged into global telecommunications networks, open and democratic, facing problems of pollution, crime, corruption, and growing demands for expensive social security benefits (Shambaugh, 1998).

Despite this growth, Taiwan had avoided social pathologies widespread in the west. Now, however, problems are emerging such as youth alienation, some crime, a small drug culture, rising divorce rates and more single parent families and trends toward unequal wealth and income distribution (Mayer, 1996). Taiwan faces two principal challenges: structural adjustments to maintain international competitiveness and comparative advantages and diversifying the technological base. A dynamic and affluent society with a dominant middle class, Taiwan is in search of greater freedoms and an improved quality of life (Shambaugh, 1998).

Democratically, life expectancy has risen and Taiwan has the highest divorce rate in Asia. The women have enjoyed substantial occupational mobility and have moved into virtually all industries and occupations. It has also enjoyed greater access to tertiary education and particularly foreign university education. Taiwan's population is one of the best-educated in Asia (Shambaugh, 1998).

Health Implication for Families and Those with Disable Child

Social Change and Family Coping

Political, economic, and demographic changes have complicated the family policy as society evolves into a multiracial, multicultural, and multilingual society. The philosophical and policy trends of de-institutionalization and normalization encourage families to raise children with developmental disabilities at home. In 1994, Executive Yuan and the Ministry of Interior reported over 90% of elderly persons in Taiwan with functional impairments are cared for by their families (Directorate-General of Budget, 1994; Directorate-General of Budget Accounting and Statistic, 1994). Due to the aging society, the parents with disabled children don't have enough time to care for the older parents who also need attention. So the social system has to develop a new program for the elderly persons.

Health Insurance Financial

The Taiwan government has instituted a national health insurance. The health care system has changed or needed replacement with some respite services for taking care of the chronically ill, disabled, or aging families. Administration, education, technical training, and research must be evolved to family health care. Healthy families could decrease social problems such as violence, drug abuse, divorce, crime, et cetera that would help to maintain international competitiveness, concern with microenvironment and develop family resources for keeping peaceful as well as decrease government or private health care spending. The social service could extend to care for the minority population such as the disabled. Multicultural, multi-language, and multi-dimensions training for the nurse profession become important in family health care.

Cultural Influence on Health Beliefs

The balance of yin and yang, or hot and cold, is one of the most important concepts in the philosophies of Confucism and Taoism. The other theory of five basic forces in the individual and universal world is metal, wood, water, fire, and earth. These concepts imply that the human being and nature are interrelated and interdependent to maintain harmony. The harmony theory, including the concepts of yin and yang and five basic forces, is important in understanding the philosophy of health and illness in Chinese culture. To re-establish the harmonious state, traditional Chinese medicine uses herbs and food to correct the disturbance and imbalance in the body systems. People in Taiwan prefer to receive Western medicine for treating acute illnesses, but in the recovery stage, they prefer to use traditional Chinese medicine to help patients restore energy and balance their body system.

According to the Buddhist philosophy of life, life is pain and suffering because of ignorance and desires. Disability is derived from the consequence of deeds done in previous lives and is associated with evil spirits. Individuals have to tolerate and accept the uncomfortable signs and symptoms associated with disability, which are viewed as the consequence of actions in a previous existence. Therefore, when a child gets a disability, both the child and family have to undergo treatment and tolerate the pain and discomforts together. In addition, they believe uncomfortable symptoms and signs relate to evil spirits or Karma. Therefore, parents take their disabled child to a temple and ask for forgiveness and purification and for an exorcism. A special charm related to a blessing from Buddha might be given to the sick child for the purpose of keeping the evil spirits away from the disable child.

Implications for Nursing Practice and Research

The conflict of creative life in human society for Taiwanese's women with a disabled child may derive from complying with Chinese life philosophies and modernism. Most women could adapt from the sacrifice associated with disabilities with resources from religion, folk belief, or social support. In addition, the women accept exhausting their energy to take care of the child; they need to participate in the religious or Chinese pattern of ritual, and respect the aged parents.

Problem solving, communication, role change, behavior control, and affective responsiveness and involvement may become the criteria for evaluating family strength. The Family Assessment Device has been used in identifying clinical and non-clinical families' adaptation; and another family functioning or family resiliency scales could help to find the problem family. Nurse professionals can develop the family strategy and policy by analyzing social system changes that influence family structure and women's role changes as well as the impact on the health care system. It is important to coordinate the family's energies to cope with the real or potential problems, social value evolution and economical vibration for making social security benefits.

There is little research in nursing that considers the family in Taiwan. Yi (1993) reviewed the articles about family studies in Taiwan, publications on family structure, family relations and women's family status that stand out as the most studied among family sociologists. The family life cycle is recognized as an important concept in teaching. The concept of roles is widely used in the women's family status literature, no single theoretical perspective can be identified as dominant in current family studies in Taiwan.

Continuing research related to family care would focus on the cultural impacts and family change corresponding to social change, comparing studies of Chinese families in different societies such as Hong Kong, Singapore and The People's Republic of China; as well as the difference between rural and urban communities.

The growth of female education achievement has profound affects on occupational and family structures. Because large numbers of married women with above-average education are entering the labor force, and there is a changing role of the employed women, it is necessary to explore the sex-role attitudes and norms to understand their family organization as well as their inputs in the work field.

Family theory should be applied to family health care to deal with family demands. Family research has to consider historical, social and philosophical changes that influence the nursing practice and national health insurance. Then, nurse professionals can make decisions on the prioritizing responsibilities and participate in making policy.

References

Adrian, S. (2002). Disability defined. *Psychology Today 35,34.*

Alcantara, M. A., Garcia-Cavazos, R., Hernandez, U. E., Gonzalez-del Angel, A., Carnevale, A., & Orozco, L. (2001). Carrier detection and prenatal molecular diagnosis in a Duchenne muscular dystrophy family without any affected relative available. *Annales de Genetique., 44*(3), 149-153.

Appleton, R. E., & Nicolaides, P. (1995). Early diagnosis of Duchenne muscular dystrophy. *Lancet, 345*, 1243-1244.

Bakker, J. P. J., de Groot, I. J. M., Beelen, A., & Lankhorst, G. J. (2002). Predictive factors of cessation of ambulation in patients with Duchenne muscular dystrophy. *American Journal Physical Medical Rehabilitation, 81*, 906-912.

Botvin, M. J. G., Radford, L. M., & Neumann, E. M. (1984). Psychosocial aspects of death and dying in Duchenne muscular dystrophy. *Archieve of Physical Medical Rehabilitation, 65*, 79-82.

Bothwell, J. E., Dooley, J. M., Gordon, K. E., MacAuley, A., Camfield, P. R., & MacSween, J. (2002). Duchenne muscular dystrophy: Parental perceptions. *Clinical Pediatrics, 41*(2), 105-109.

Bradley, D. M., Parsons, E. P., & Clarke, A. J. (1993). Experience with screening newborns for Duchenne muscular dystrophy in Wales. *British Medical Journal, 306*, 357-360.

Buchanan, D., LaBarbera, C., Roelofs, R., & Olson, W. (1979). Reactions of families to children with Duchenne muscular dystrophy. *General Hospital Psychiatry, 3*, 262-269.

Cambridge, M. A. (1995). Negotiating the meaning of women's work, family, and kinship in urban Taiwan in Harvard studies on Taiwan Vol I, *Fairbank Center for East Asian Research* (pp. 271-285).

Cause of death statistics (2001). Department of health Taiwan, R. O. C. Retrieved December, 2, 2002, from the World Wide Web: http://www.doh.gov.tw/statistics/data

Chan, H. S., & Yang, Y. (1995). The development of social welfare in Taiwan. *Free China Journal, 3*(March), 4.

Chen, C. (1991, September, 15). Court sentence on teachers revives old controversy. *China Post.* pp. 9.

Chen, J. Y., Chen, S. S., Jong, Y. J., Yang, Y. H., & Lue, Y. J. (2003, April 10-12). *Psychosocial stress and coping strategies of parents with Duchenne muscular*

dystrophy children during the middle stage. Paper presented at the 36th Annual
Communicating Nursing Research Conference & 17th Annual Win Assembly,
Scottsdale Arizona.

Chen, J. Y., Chen, S. S., Jong, Y. J., & Yang, Y. H. (2002). *The impact for the parents with
Ducehnne muscular dystrophy children.*Unpublished manuscript.

Chen, J. Y., & Jong, Y. J. (2006). A stress model for parents of children with Duchenne
muscular dystrophy. *The Journal of Nursing (Chinese), 53*(3), 44-51.

Cheng, J. (1995). More senior citizens, fewer kids. *Free China Review, 45*(12), 42-46.

Chiu, K. (1996). Job equity act given the green light. *Free China Journal, 19*(April), 4.

Chang, M. C., Freedman, R., & Sun, T. H. (1981). Trends in fertility, family size preferences,
and family planning practice: Taiwan, 1961-1980. *Studies in Family Planning, 12*,
211-228.

Chu, H. Y. (1992). The impact of different religions on the Chinese family in Taiwan. In J. C.
Hsieh & Y. C. Chuang (Eds.), *The Chinese family and its ritual behavior.* Taipei,
Republic of China: Institute of Ethnology, Academia Sinica.

Chu, H. Y., & Wen, C. I. (1975). Value change in modernization processes: a comparative
study of three Taipei communities. *TW, 12*(5), 1-14.

Chuang, Y. C. (1992). Family structure and reproductive patterns in a Taiwan fishing village.
In J. C. Hsieh & Y. C. Chuang (Eds.), *The Chinese family and its ritual behaviors* (pp.
128-161). Taipei: Institute of Ethnology, Academia Sinica.

Cohen, O., Slonim, I., Finzi, R., & Leichtentritt, R. D. (2002). Family resilience: Israeli
mothers' perspectives. *American Journal of Family Therapy, 30*, 173-187.

Dean, K. (1993). *Taoist ritual and popular cults of southeast China.* Princeton, New Jersey:
Princeton University.

Department of Health, Taiwan R. O. C. (2001). Crude birth rates, crude death rates and
natural increase rates, Taiwan area, 1962-2001. Retrieved January 23, 2003, from
http://www.doh.gov.tw/statistic/data

Directorate- General of Budget, Accounting and Statistics. (1993). Taipei: Executive Yuan,
Social Indicator in Taiwan Area of Republic of China.

Directorate-General of Budget, A. a. S. (1994). *Report on the old status survey: Taiwan Area
R. O. C.* Taipei, Taiwan: Executive Yuan & Ministry of Interior, ROC.

Directorate-General of Budget Accounting and Statistic. (1994). *Report on the old status survey: Taiwan Area R. O. C.* Taipei, Taiwan: Executive Yuan & Ministry of Interior, ROC.

Emery, A. E. H. (2002). The muscular dystrophies. *Lancet, 359*(9307), 687.

Emery, A. E. H. (1993). *Duchenne muscular dystrophy* (2 ed.). Oxford: Oxford Medical Publish.

Epstein, N. B., Bishop, D. S., Ryan, C. E., Miller, I. W., & Keitner, G. I. (1993). The McMaster Model: View of healthy family functioning. In F. Walsh (Ed.), *Normal family processes* (pp. 138-160). New York: Guilford.

Failla, S., & Jones, L. C. (1991). Families of children with developmental disabilities: An examination of family hardiness. *Research in Nursing & health, 14,* 41-50.

Farris, C. S. (1993). Women, work, and child care in Taiwan: Changing family dynamics in a chinese society. *American Asian Review, 11*(3), 134-151.

Firth, M. A., Gardner-Medwin, D., Hosking, G., & Wilkinson, E. (1983). Interviews with parents of boys suffering from Duchenne muscular dystrophy. *Development Medicine and Child Neurology, 25,* 466-471.

Fitzpatrick, C., & Barry, C. (1990). Cultural differences in family communication about Duchenne muscular dystrophy. *Developmental Medicine and Child Neurology, 32,* 967-973.

Francke, U., Ochs, H. D., de Martinville, B., Giacalone, J., Lindgren, V., Disteche, C., et al. (1985). Minor Xp21 chromosome deletion in a male associated with expression of Duchenne muscular dystrophy, chronic granulomatous disease, retinitis pigmentosa, and McLeod syndrome. *American Journal Human Genetic, 37*(250-267).

Freedman, M. (1958). Lineage organization in southeastern China. *London school of economics monographs on social anthropology, 18.*

Freedman, M. (1979). The politics of an old state: A view from the Chinese lineage in G. W. In G. W. Skinner (Ed.), *The study of Chinese society: Essays by Maurice Freedman.* Stanford: Stanford University.

Gagliardi, B. A. (1991). The family's experience of living with a child with Duchenne muscular dystrophy. *Applied Nursing Research, 4*(4), 159-164.

Geography (2002a). Retrieved Nov, 6, 2002, from the World Wide Web: http://www.marimari.com/content/taiwan/general_info/geography/geography.html

Geography (2002b). Retrieved Nov 6, 2002, from the World Wide Web:
http://www.maramari.com/content/taiwan/general_inf/geography/geography.html

Gold, T. B. (1996 in China Quartely). Taiwan society at the Fin de Siecle. In D. Shambaugh
(Ed.), *Contemporary Taiwan* (pp. 47-70). Oxford: Clarendon.

Gottlieb, A. (1998). Single mother of children with disabilities: the role of sense of coherence
in managing multiple challenges. In J. E. Fromer (Ed.), *Stress, coping, and health in
families: sense of coherence and resilience* (pp. 189-206). Thousand Oaks, CA: Sage.

Greenhalgh, S. (1984). Networks and their nodes: urban society on Taiwan. *The China
Quartely, 99*, 529-552.

Habito, M. R. (2002). The Taipei, Taiwan, Museum of world religions. *Buddhist-Christian
Studies*, 203-205.

Hoffman, E. P., Brown, R. H. J., & Kunkel, L. M. (1987). Dystrophin: The protein product of
the Duchenne muscular dystrophy locus. *Cell, 51*, 919-928.

Holroyd, J., & Guthrie, D. (1986). Family stress with chronic childhood illness: Cystic
fibrosis, neuromuscular disease, and renal disease. *Journal Clinical Psychology, 42*(4),
552-561.

Huang, L., & Dai, Y. (1998). Psychosocial impact of muscular dystrophy on mothers
[Chinese]. *Journal of Nursing Research (China), 6*(2), 137-151.

Hsieh, J. C. (1992). Meal rotation. In J. C. Hsieh & Y. C. Chuang (Eds.), *The Chinese family
and its ritual behaviors* (pp. 70-83). Taipei: Institute of Ethnology, Academia Sinica.

Jordan, D. K. (1972). *Gods, ghosts, and ancestors: the folk religion of a Taiwanese village.*
Berkeley, Los Angeles: University of California.

Kilmer, D. D., Abresch, R. T., & Fowler, W. M. J. (1993). Serial manual muscle testing in
Duchenne muscular dystrophy. *Archieve Physical Medicine Rehabilitation, 74*, 1168-
1171.

Koenig, M., Hoffman, E. P., Bertelson, C. J., Monaco, A. P., Feener, C., & Kunkel, L. M.
(1987). Complete cloning of the Duchenne muscular dystrophy (DMD) cDNA and
preliminary genomic organization of the DMD gene in normal and affected
individuals. *Cell, 50*, 509-517.

Laing, N. G. (1993). Molecular genetics and genetic counseling for Duchenne /Becker
muscular dystrophy. In T. Patridge (Ed.), *Molecular and cell biology of muscular
dystrophy* (pp. 37-84). London: Chapman & Hall.

Lin, D. (1995). ROC wins the World's applause for strides in family planning. *Free China Journal, 14*(July), 4.

Lin, M. (1990). Greater demand for size XL. *Free China Review, 40*(1), 49-51.

Liu, P. (1995). Hassles with health care. *Free China Review, 45*(4), 52-58.

Long-Term Care Profession Association of ROC. (1997). *The list of registered long-term care services in Taiwan.* Taipei, Taiwan. (in Chinese): Long-Term Care Profession Association of ROC.

Lue, Y. J., Chen, S. S., Jong, Y. J., & Lin, Y. T. (1993). Investigation of activity of daily living performance in patients with Duchenne Muscular Dystrophy. *Kaohsiung Journal Medical Science, 9,* 351-360.

Making policy to encourage fertility (2002). Chinese Time Newspaper. Retrieved December 2, 2002, from the World Wide Web: http://www.yahoo.com.tw

Margalit, M., Raviv, A., & Ankonina, D. B. (1992). Coping and coherence among parents with disabled children. *Journal of Clinical Child Psychology, 21,* 202-209.

Marsh, R. M. (1996). *Taiwan in the modern world: The great transformation: Social change in Taipei, Taiwan since the 1960s.* Armonk, New York: M. E. Sharpe.

Marsh, R. M., & Hsu, C. K. (1994). Modernization and changes in extended kinship in Taipei, Taiwan: 1963-1991. In P. L. Lin & K. W. Mei & H. C. Peng (Eds.), *Marriage and the family in Chinese societies* (pp. 53-78). Indianapolis: University of Indianapolis.

Nereo, N. E., Fee, R. J., & Hinton, V. J. (2003). Parental stress in mothers of boys with Ducehnne muscular dystrophy. *Journal of Pediatric Psychology, 28,* 473-484.

Nereo, N. E., & Hinton, V. J. (2003). Three wishes and psychological functioning in boys with Duchenne muscular dystrophy. *Developmental and Behavioral Pediatrics, 24*(2), 96-103.

Ng, C. Y., Phillips, D. R., & Lee, K. M. (2002). Persistence and challenges to filial piety and informal support of older personsm in a modern Chinese society: A case study in Tuen Mun, Hong Kong. *Journal of Aging Studies, 16,* 135-153.

Parent Project Muscular Dystrophy. (2002). The basics of muscular dystrophy and beyond: Progression of Duchenne MD. Retrieved December 12, 2003, from www.parentprojectmd.org/aboutdmd/basics/progress.html

Patterson, J. M. (2002). *Promoting resilience in families experiencing stress.* University of Minnesota, School of Public Health Retrieved August 6, 2002, from http://www..epi.umi.edu/epi_pages/Syllabi/reading2.html

Patterson, J. M., & McCubbin, H. I. (1983). Chronic illness: Family stress and coping. In H. I. McCubbin (Ed.), *Stress and the family: Volume II: Coping with catastrophe* (pp. 21-36). New York: Brunner/Mazel.

Rideau, Y., Duport, G., Delaubier, A., Guillon, C., Renardel-Irani, A., & Bach, J. R. (1995). Early treatment to preserve quality of locomotion for children with Duchenne muscular dystrophy. *Seminar in Neurology, 15*, 9-17.

Roland, E. H. (2000). Muscular dystrophy. *Pediatric in Review, 21*(7), 233.

Shambaugh, D. (1998). *Contemporary Taiwan*. Oxford: Clearendon Press.

Shih, K. (2002). *Family and life course studies: long term research goals*. Institute of Sociology, Academia Sinica. Retrieved November, 3, 2002, from the World Wide Web: http://140.109.196.186/life/myweb2/english/introduction.html

Siegel, I. M., Davidson, H., Kornfeld, M., & McCready, W. C. (1983). Coping with muscular dystrophy: Psychosocial correlates of adaptation. *Muscle and Nerve, 6*, 607-609.

Siciliano, G., Tessa, A., Renna, M., Manca, M. L., Mancuso, M., & Murri, L. (1999). Epidemiology of dystrophinopathies in North-West Tuscany: A molecular genetics-based revisitation. *Clinical Genetics, 56*, 51-58.

Smith, D. C. (1977-1979). *Higher education in Taiwan: The Confucius-Dewey Synthesis*: Pacific Cultural Foundation: Academic Books Co.

Smith, R. A., Williams, D. K., Sibert, J. R., & Harper, P. S. (1990). Attitude of mothers to neonatal screening for DMD. *British Medicine Journal, 28*, 300.

Taiwan geography (2001). Federation of American Scientistics. Retrieved Nov 6, 2002, from the World Wide Web: http://www.fas.org/man/dod-101/ops/taiwan_people.html

Taiwan geography (2002). Retrieved Nov 6, 2002, from the World Wide Web: http://www.fas.org/man/dod-101/ops/taiwan_geohtm

Taiwan introduction 2000 (2000). Retrieved 2002, Nov 6, from the World Wide Web: http://www.photius.com.com/wfb2000/countries/taiwan/taiwan_introduction.html

Teta, J. A. (1971). *Taiwan in picture*. New York: Sterling, Publishing.

Thompson, R. J. J., Zeman, J. L., Fanurik, D., & Sirotkin-Roses, M. (1992). The role of parent stress and coping and family functioning in parent and child adjustment to Duchenne muscular dystrophy. *Journal of Clinical Psychology, 48*, 11-19.

Thornton, A., Chang, M. C., & Sun, T. H. (1984). Social and economic change, intergenerational relationships and family formation in Taiwan. *Demography, 21*(4), 475-499.

Thornton, A., & Lin, H. S. (1994). *Socail change and the family in Taiwan.* Chicago: University of Chicago.

TMDA. (2002). TMDA bulletin: 019. Retrieved January 23, 2003, from tmda.adsldns.org

Traditional Chinese culture in Taiwan: Philosophy (2002). Retrieved September 21, 2002, from the World Wide Web: http://www.housetoncul.org/culdir/phil/phil.htm

Vignos, P. J. J., Wagner, M. B., Karlinchak, B., & Katirji, B. (1996). Evaluation of a program for long-term treatment of Duchenne muscular dystrophy, experience at the University Hospital of Cleveland. *Journal of Bone and Joint Surgery, 78A*(12), 1844-1852.

Walsh, F. (1998). *Strengthening family resilience.* New York: Guilford Press.

Whyte, M. K. (1992). *From arranged marriages to love matches in urban China.* Hong Kong: HongKong Institute of Asia-Pacific Studies, Chinese University of Hong Kong.

Wolf, M. (1972). *Women and the family in rural Taiwan.* Standford, California: Standford University.

Yi, C. C. (1993). Studying social change: the case of Taiwanese family sociologists. *Current Sociology, 41*, 41-67.

Yi, C. C., & Chien, W. Y. (2002). The linkage between work and family: Female's employment patterns in three Chinese societies. *Journal of Comparative Family Studies, 33*, 451-474.

Yuan, Y. (1993). Small is still big. *Free China Review, 43*(11), 5-12.

Yun, E. (1993). Child care choices. *Free China Review, 43*(11), 20-24.

Part Two

Asking Compelling Clinical Questions

Resilience in Families of Children with Disabilities

Introduction

More than 10 million children in America have a developmental disability and as many as 50% of children with disabilities are not identified until school age. Having a chronic disease increases one's risk for secondary conditions (Adrian, 2002). Disability means an incapacity or disqualification. A child with a disability means the child is deprived of physical and/or mental abilities. Disabling conditions are life-long and often require services from many agencies that increase financial costs, caregiver burden, and social isolation, as well as restricting life-styles and career opportunities (Failla & Jones, 1991; Gottlieb, 1998; Patterson & McCubbin, 1983).

The reciprocal impacts on the families are circular and continuous (Patterson, 2002). The sacrifices associated with chronic disease and disabilities are not temporary but become a way of life for the whole family with a disabled child. The family may have already depleted family energy and resources when the chronic condition deteriorates.The transition of a child with disabilities affects and is affected by the family social system.

The philosophical and policy trends of de-institutionalization and normalization encourage families to raise children with developmental disabilities at home. Advances in medical science and changes in public policy have resulted in more disabled children supported in the community and at home. As more disabled children stay at home, families must become more diverse in their skills to meet the challenges and the special risks. In addition, the nation evolves into a multiracial, multicultural, and multilingual society (Braverman, 2001; Wisensale, 1993). As a result, family issues surrounding the adaptation of coping with a child with a disability must be viewed in light of these changes.

Four important trends in a socio-historical context are: "diverse family forms," "changing gender roles and relations," "cultural diversity and socioeconomic disparity," and "varying and expanded family life cycle course" (Walsh, 1998, p.26). Despite transitions in their structure, families remain the most basic unit of society. There is encouraging evidence that research and resulting programs can contribute to the strength and resilience of all families.

More recently, attention has been focused on how a family copes with and adapts to a very difficult situation in an attempt to promote health and well being; to maintain the family's stability, social support, integration, and self-esteem; and to communicate with other families and medical teams. However, the slow and arduous illness course that can lead to parental strain or adaptation has received little attention in nursing.

Researchers have observed that some individuals who experience a high degree of life stress remain healthy. They become actively involved in events, viewing them as meaningful, maintaining hope and attachment, and finding social support. Life changes are viewed as opportunities for growth and development (Failla & Jones, 1991). This phenomenon can explain which resilience processes that adaptive families have developed to deal with their problems and cope effectively (Cohen, Slonim, Finzi, & Leichtentritt, 2002). However, a few articles in nursing applied the resilience model to evidence family adaptation of disabilities.

Family resilience is an important indication of overall adjustment and adaptation in the family with a disabled child. Exploring and developing the knowledge related to family resilience will help to develop and maintain the capacity of a family to be resilient, and will help to understand the influence of factors on family adaptation and resilience. The purpose of this paper is to explore the phenomenon of family resilience specifically on a disabled family. The first part defines resilience and family resilience, and their attributes. The second part reviews the literature associated with the concept of the family resilience in order to address the factors of family resilience and to understand how they contribute to the family resilience process. It is important to look at factors contributing to family resilience that helps to develop the variables of an empirical study and may help to design programs that promote adjustment and adaptation of the families of the disabled child. The third component reviews the research to identify the indicators of concepts, to locate measurement tools, and to analyze and critique the state of the science on the related research. The researcher explains the importance of establishing the body of knowledge of family resilience in nursing to facilitate and to expand family center care. In summary, the researcher identifies the implications of the various studies on nursing practice and education and suggests the future studies based on the gaps of knowledge in previous research.

Where Do We Go on This Idea?

Family-center nursing care is not only to promote individual health but also to uphold and maintain family strengths to help families in keeping with community supports, and to achieve a realistic appraisal of what is the best fit for them in their specific situation. So, the nursing professional not only studies individual resilience but also is concerned with family resilience for the family with a disabled child. Finally, the research finds the framework of family resilience to be measured and compared the differences of the models. Then explore how resilient families with a child with a chronic condition can balance the demands of each other in the family, maintain social integration, a positive outlook, commitment, family boundaries, flexibility, time together, and connectedness; and to develop communication competence and open emotional expression; to collaborate relationships with professionals (collaborative problem solving), to make meaning of adversity, and the flexibility to shift roles and provide support.

What is the body knowledge in the phenomena?

Theoretical of Framework

The Resiliency Model of Family Stress, Adjustment, and Adaptation is based on (a) Hill's (1949, 1958) ABCX family crisis model, (b) the Double ABCX model: Family Adaptation (McCubbin & Patterson, 1981, 1983), (c) the FAAR: Family Adjustment and Adaptation Response model (McCubbin, McCubbin, Thompson, & Thompson, 1998; Patterson, 1988), and (d) the Typology of Family Adjustment and Adaptation (McCubbin & McCubbin, 1987). The Hill's (1949, 1958) ABCX family crisis model states that A (stressor and hardships) interacting with B (resources) and C (the family's definition of the stressor) as the critical variables produces X (family crisis) (McCubbin, McCubbin, Thompson, & Thompson, 1998; McCubbin, 1993). The Double ABCX model focus on the factors affecting family adaptation: XX (Family adaptation), AA (family demands: pile-up), BB (family adaptive resources), and CC (family definition and meaning). The FAAR: Family Adjustment and Adaptation Response model emphasized the processes of balancing demands (stressor and strain) and capabilities (resources and coping behaviors) (McCubbin, McCubbin et al., 1998; Patterson, 1988) and is arbitrated by the meanings the family attributes to what is happening to them. Over time the family passes through repeated cycles of adjustment and adaptation (Patterson, 2002). The Typology of Family Adjustment and Adaptation (McCubbin & McCubbin, 1987) emphasized the importance of the family's established patterns of functioning and the family appraisal processes including family values, beliefs, and expectations and focused on family change and adaptation overtime (Kosciulek, McCubbin, & McCubbin, 1993). All these models focused on a stressor, family resources, and family appraisal of the situation, family coping patterns, and problem-solving abilities to maintain function during dealing with stressors.

McCubbin and McCubbin (1993) established the Resiliency Model of Family Stress, Adjustment, and Adaptation. The model includes two phases: adjustment and adaptation. The adjustment phase is composed of interacting components that shape the family process and outcomes: (a) the stressor; (b) the family's vulnerability; (c) the family typology of functioning; (d) the family's resources; (e) the family's appraisal of the stressor; and (f) the family's problem-solving and coping strategies. These components interact with one another to determine the level of adjustment in the family. If the family is successful in its response to the stressor, the family passes through the situation and produces a positive outcome called bonadjustment (McCubbin & McCubbin, 1993). In illness situations, especially chronic illness or disability, however, hardships are often numerous and severe, demanding more changes in the family system, and the family may experience maladjustment and a resulting state of crisis. Family crisis is a period of family disorganization, family disharmony, and imbalance in the system, which moves to the onset of the adaptation phase. In the adaptation phase, interacting components that operate include (a) the pileup of demands on or in the family system created by the illness, family life-cycle change, and unresolved strains; (b) the family typology, determined in part by newly instituted patterns of family functioning and retained established patterns of functioning (regenerative or resiliency); (c) the family's resources; (d) social support from extended family, friends, and the community; (e) a situational appraisal; (f) the family's schema appraisal and the family's meaning; and (g) the family's problem solving and coping. Family adaptation is the outcome of the family's efforts over time to meet both the needs of individual and family members to achieve their 7personal growth and also the functioning of the family system and its transitions with the community (McCubbin & McCubbin, 1993).

The Model assists nurse professionals in assessing family functioning and intervening in the family system to facilitate both family adjustment and family adaptation, and to determine what family types, capabilities, and strengths are needed. But all the articles do not include both phases. This limitation makes it necessary for the researcher to find another theory or concept to analyze and compare with the family resilience model. In strengthening family functioning nursing professionals can use the model for designing the programs and studies.

What is Resilience?

Definition of Resiliency

Over the past 2 decades, the definition of resilience is the ability to withstand and rebound from adversity that has become an important concept. Resilience is a manifestation of competence despite exposure to significant stressors. Cohen, and his colleagues (2002) stated, "resilience processes contribute to family dynamics and the family's abilities to cope effectively and adapt in crises" (p.183). Resilience involves a dynamic process encompassing positive adaptation within the context of significant adversity (Luthar, cicchetti, & Becker, 2000). Early studies focused on personal traits associated with resilience, or hardiness, reflecting the dominant cultural ethos of the rugged individual (Walsh, 2002). Resilience and vulnerability are often viewed as opposite poles of a continuum reflecting susceptibility to adverse consequences or benign consequences upon exposure to higher risk circumstance (Anthony, 1987). Rutter (1990, p. 181) defined resilience as a positive pole of ubiquitous phenomenon of individual difference in people's response to stress and adversity.

Resilience is derived from the individual's perception and experience. Examining definitions of resilience in dictionaries and articles, most authors used the terms "ability," "power," or "capacity" to recover, overcome, resist, or bounce back from misfortune and adversity (Walsh, 2002). Some used "change," "resist," or "cultivate strengths" to positively meet the challenge of life (Brown, 1993; Flexner & Hauck, 1993; Robison & Davidson, 1996; Thames & Thomason, 2000). Luthar, Cicchetti, and Becker (2000) presented resilience as "a dynamic process encompassing positive adaptation within the context of significant adversity" (p. 543). More recently, researchers have used the term "adapt" to relate the concept of resilience to healthy development or conditions.

Wolin and Wolin (1993) constructed the traits of resilience that include insight, independence, initiative, relationship, humor, creativity, and morality. Resilience is not simply the ability to cope with everyday stress, but includes confidence, cooperation, hard work, and forgiveness that increases the family's well being (Thames et al., 2000, ¶ 1). Resilience applied to family helps families to be resistant to disruption in the face of change and adapt in the face of the crisis, offers families an opportunity to change in constructive ways and to strengthen family bonds (Benard, 2001).

Family-center nursing care is not only to promote individual health but also to uphold and maintain family strengths, to help families connect with community supports, and to achieve a realistic appraisal of what is the best fit for them in their specific situation. The health provider not only study individual resilience but also is concerned with family resilience for the family with a disabled child. Finally, the research finds the measurements relating to framework of family resilience and compared the differences of the models.

What is Family Resilence?

Family resilience is the family's ability to exhibit strengths to positively face the challenge of life. The definition of family resilience derives from a resiliency model of family stress, adjustment, and adaptation. McCubbin and McCubbin (1988) indicated that family resilience is "a characteristic, dimension, and property of families which helps families to be resistant to disruption in the face of change and adaptive in the face of crisis situations" (p. 247). Walsh (1998) identified three domains of family resilience, "family belief system, organizational pattern, and communicational process" (p. 24). The first belief systems include "making meaning of adversity, positive outlook, and transcendence and spirituality"; the second organizational patterns include "flexibility, connectedness, social and economic resources"; the third communication processes include "clarity, open emotional expression, and collaborative problem solving" (p. 133). The nine categories are clarified in the three domains to guide in three different approaches in the study. The model has been to be applied in nursing practice and research. Resilient families can positively respond to the interactive combination of risk and recovery factors, and share beliefs or feelings (Hawley & De Haan, 1996).

Well-adjusted families returned to a steady state of functioning after the changes occurred. Of the more recent measures of family functioning (3 observational, 22 questionnaires, 1 interview, and 2 Q-sorts), 24 focused on the entire family, 2 on the marital dyad, and 1 on the sibling dyad. The most frequently assessed dimensions of family functioning include cohesion, the ability to grow, adaptation, communication, affective involvement, and control (Touliator, Perlmutter, & Straus, 1990). Sawin & Hawigan (1994) reviewed three categories of family functioning instrument they can be used to predict phenomena associated with family functioning.

In illness situations, especially chronic illness or disability, however, hardships are often numerous and severe, demanding more changes in the family system, and the family may experience maladjustment and a resulting state of crisis. Family crisis is a period of family disorganization, family disharmony, and imbalance in the system, which moves to the onset of the adaptation phase. In the adaptation phase, interacting components that operate include (a) the pileup of demands on or in the family system created by the illness, family life-cycle change, and unresolved strains; (b) the family typology, determined in part by newly instituted patterns of family functioning and retained established patterns of functioning; (c) the family's resources; (d) social support from extended family, friends, and the community; (e) a situational appraisal; (f) the family's schema appraisal and the family's meaning; and (g) the family's problem solving and coping. Family adaptation is the outcome of the family's efforts over time to meet both the needs of individual and family members to achieve their personal growth and also the functioning of the family system and its transitions with the community (McCubbin & McCubbin, 1993).

Kazak's (1992) indicated research on the adaptation of families of children with disabilities had profited from incorporating aspects of social ecology theory, family systems theory, and family stress theory, quality and nature of the family environment (including the marital relationship, family cohesiveness and adaptability, and parenting styles, and the quantity and efficacy of informal support systems utilized by families helped to explain variation in parental and family adaptation to a typical parenting experience (cited in Hauser-Cram et al., 1998).

Dyson (1997) found that although fathers and mothers of children with disabilities did not differ in levels of parental stress, social support, or family functioning, parental stress was related to family problems due to the child's special needs, to the family's emotional climate and to parents' pessimism concerning the child's future. Strauss-Leonard formed that only two typologies recognized a disabled form of the open type in their original formulation equated the normal families or healthy family functioning.

Researchers have found increasing evidence that the same adversity can result in different outcomes. Early studies focused on personal traits associated with resilience, or hardiness, reflecting the dominant cultural ethos of rugged individual. As research extended beyond situations of parental mental illness or maltreatment to multiple adverse conditions, resilience has involved individual, family, and larger sericulture influences. Family assessment measures play an important role in the identification of strengths and needs relates to an overall vision or philosophy of family functioning. There is a need for a multidimensional framework that will facilitate the assessment of family functioning along several dimensions at the same time to evaluate the DMD family function and family resiliency.

From a family perspective, resilience may refer to the adaptability that Hill in 1949 found to be functional for families in withstanding stress over time. The concept of family resilience offers a useful framework to identify key processes that enable families to surmount crises and persistent stresses. A resiliency-based approach aims to identify and fortify key interactional processes that enable families to withstand and rebound from the disruptive challenges they face of crisis situations (Walsh, 1996).

The focus of the resiliency model is to understand those family strengths and capabilities that buffer the family from the disruptions associated with normative family transitions and non-normative stressors. Strong families are able to adapt to changing circumstances and have a positive attitude towards the challenges of family life. Key components of the resiliency model that assist in explaining family behavior in response to stressors are the family's resources, the family's appraisal of their situation, and family adaptation (McCubbin et al., 1996). Family resources are potential capabilities the family has available for meeting demands (Olson, Russell, & Sprenkle, 1983; Olson, Sprenkle, & Russell, 1979), and social support (McCubbin et al., 1996). Family cohesion is defined as the emotional bonding members have with each other and the degree of personal autonomy experienced in the family (Olson et al., 1979). Family adaptability is defined as the ability of the family to change its power structure, roles, and rules in response to situational and developmental stress.

What Factors are Contributing to Family Resilience?

Family protective factors and family recovery factors are the two components of family resilience, which are viewed as positive counterparts to family vulnerability and family crisis (McCubbin, McCubbin, Thompson, Han, & Allen, 1997). The protective factors include family hardiness, family communication, financial management, support network, family bonding, and family time (Family resiliency, 2002). The recovery factors include family support, problem solving coping skills, family optimism and mastery, family advocacy, family meaning, and family schema (McCubbin et al., 1997). In addition, individual resilience factors and the traits of resilience (McCubbin & McCubbin, 1993) will help to promote the relationship of families and will help to develop the family resilience.

What Do We Know the Concept?

Related Concepts and Measurements

The researcher depended on the nursing process to explore resilience in family with a disabled child. There are five key components to evaluate: (a) family stressors and family strains; (b) family resources; (c) family problem solving and coping; (d) family appraisal, family coherence, and family schema; and (e) family adaptation.

McCubbin, Thompson, and McCubbin (1996) defined family stressor as a demand placed on the family that produces changes in the family system (e.g., life cycle, family boundary, family type). The stressor may threaten the stability of the family units or place significant demands on the family's resources and capabilities. A family type is a set of attributes that can predict and discern patterns of family functioning (McCubbin et al., 1996). The researchers usually used Family Inventory of Life Events and Changes (McCubbin et al., 1996) to measure the family stressors and strains.

McCubbin et al. (1996) describe family resource as a family's capabilities and strengths to resist a crisis and promote family resilience to establish patterns of function and achieve harmony and balance. Hardiness contains three components: control, commitment, and challenge. Family Hardiness Index, the Family Inventory of Resources for Management, and the Family Time and Routines Index were often used to measure the characteristics of hardiness as a stress resistance and adaptation resource that refers to the internal strengths and durability of the family unit (McCubbin, Thompson, & McCubbin, 1996).

These terms "family problem solving and coping" indicate the action that reflect a family's ability to deal with the stressor and hardship to maintain or restore the family harmony and balance. Researchers often used the Coping Health Inventory for Parents, F-COPES: Family Crisis Oriented Personal Evaluation Scales, and Family Problem Solving Communication to measure the degree of the family coping strategies (McCubbin, et al., 1996).

Family appraisal is the family perception of the seriousness of a disability and its hardships. It contains family beliefs and expectations regarding disability. It was defined as a familial sense of coherence. It was measured using the Family Sense of Coherence (Antonovsky & Sourani, 1988).

Family schema is a structure of fundamental convictions, values, beliefs, and expectations (McCubbin et al., 1996; McCubbin, Thompson, Thompson, Elver, & McCubbin, 1998). A family schema includes cultural-ethical beliefs, and values. It was measured using the Family (Ethnicity) Schema Index (McCubbin, Thompson et al., 1998).

Family cohesion is defined as the emotional bonding among family members and the degree of personal autonomy experienced in the family, as well as the degree of family adaptability (Olson, Sprenkle, & Russell, 1979). Family adaptability is defined as the ability of the family system to change its power structure, roles, and rules in response to situational and developmental stress (McCubbin et al., 1996). It was measured using the Family Adaptability and Cohesion Evaluation Scale (Olson, Portner, & Bell, 1982).

Family adaptation is the outcome of the family's efforts in response to family stressors and is defined as a minimal discrepancy between demands and capabilities (McCubbin et al., 1996), and to bring a new or satisfactory level of balance, harmony, coherence, and functioning to family crisis situations (McCubbin et al., 1996). It was measured using the Family Assessment Device (Epstein, Baldwin, & Bishop, 1983).

Strength of Empirical Studies on Family Resilience

The resilience model has been studied with a number of families dealing with chronic illness, disability, adversity, and trauma. The criteria of review articles selected was based on the subject coming from a family with a disabled child, or selected because measurements were with the whole family resilience model but with a non-disabled family. The researcher depended on the relationship of predictor variables of family resiliency model to analyze and critique. Related factors of family adaptation were first analyzed. Then related factors of family function were described.

After reviewing the articles, the researcher know there are 4 factors that influence family adaptation: sense of coherence and using of resource, stress related to emotional climate and pessimism concerning the child future, social support and family strengths; and there are 3 group of factors that influence family functioning: family hardiness, family support, and family communication; family problem solving communication, family schema, and family meaning; family time together, life-style, pile-up of stressors and strains. The following discusses these factors.

61

Influence Factors Related to Family Adaptation

    Sense of coherence and use of resources

Kazak (1992) indicated that the quality and nature of the family environment and the quantity and efficacy of informal support systems utilized by families helped to explain variation in parental and family adaptation to a typical parenting experience. Bristor (1991) described that quality of the physically disabled children may depend to a large degree on the parents' ability to love the child completely. In addition, socio-economic or material resource, locus of control, self-esteem, relationship with the family and social network, and service response can provide resistance against stress (Knussen & Sloper, 1992).

Gottlieb's (1998) research has emphasized stress and coping resources in single-mother families and families of children with disabilities. In a study of 152 single mothers he found that their sense of coherence was associated with family coherence. Results revealed that if these single mothers had a strong sense of coherence and greater use of resources then they had more adaptive outcomes.

Lustig (1997) studied 116 parents of adult children with mental retardation. Results indicated that most families were resilient and functioning positive. There were positive correlations between scores on family adaptation, and social support, family sense of coherence, and family adaptability. The major contribution was to develop an empirical family typology and establish the knowledge of family sense of coherence. The weak points were the low response rate, the sampling procedure was nonrandom and cross-sectional, and the interpretation of the results should be limited to the sample examined at the time of the study.

    Stress related to emotional climate and pessimism concerning the child's future

Dyson (1997) found that although fathers and mothers of children with disabilities did not differ in levels of parental stress, social support, or family functioning; parental stress was related to family problems due to the child's special needs, to the family's emotional climate, and to parents' pessimism concerning the child's future. Simmerman and Blacher (2001) described that mothers' satisfaction with fathers' help related more strongly to indicators of family well-being than the actual extent of fathers' help.

    Social support

Judge (1998) conducted the study examining the relationship between parental perceptions of coping strategies and family strengths from 69 parents of young children with disabilities. The results showed that the use of social support was highly associated with family strengths. Additional results indicated that wishful thinking, self-blame, distancing, and self-control were negatively related to family strengths. The major contribution is that evidence provides family's informal and formal sources to strengthen family functioning. The sample size is too small to generalize the findings, and the majority of participants were Caucasian and all resided in one geographical region so results may not be applicable to families from other cultures or geographic areas.

Tak and McCubbin (2000) designed a longitudinal study with 92 families of children with a congenital heart disease. The results revealed perceived social support as a resilience factor and as well as a predictor of family coping. The limitation of the study was not used causal path analysis to explain of moderating and mediating effects.

Atkin and Ahmad (2000) interviewed 37 parents who had children with thalassemia and 25 parents who had children with a sickle cell disease. The results revealed that appropriate professional support helps to reduce stress and facilitate coping by offering information, financial, help and emotional support. Health providers can empower families to care for their disabled children by coordinate various medical care, making care accessible, and providing an appropriate service delivery system.

Bennett and Deluca (1996) used in-depth interviews of 12 parents with a disabled child to investigate the use of networks. Results showed that parents got (a) emotional support and caregiving from families and friends; (b) emotional outlet and source of information from parent groups; (c) development of ideas and actions and support from professionals. The implication is that a social network has an effect on family adaptation.

McCubbin, McCubbin, and Thompson (1993) conducted in Hawaii the impact of pressures, strengths, and capacities on family life with about 200 families including Caucasian (N=78), Asian (N=49), Hawaiian (N=37), and mixed-race families (N=36). The results showed that social support appeared to have greater explanatory power than other indexes for family adaptation; family care responsibilities appeared to have greater than other indexes effect on family maladaptation.

The major strength of the study is that it used a random digit dialing process and the sample size is enough to compare the impact of disability on families in four different races. The second strength is guided by resilience model to construct interviews and identified the reliability and validity of each psychometric measures of family adaptation. The third area of strength is evident in the two critical explanatory factors, family schema and appraisal. These two factors affect a family's adaptation. The major contribution for the professional are that they need to know how to inquire about family schema and recognize importance of family appraisal in shaping family function, adjustment, and adaptation.

Family strengths

McIntyre (2000) examined 77 mothers' role of competency-enhancing help in the adaptation process for mothers of children with special needs and found (a) higher levels of competency-enhancing help were related to greater maternal adaptation as measured by maternal sense of well-being and satisfaction with family functioning; (b) competency-enhancing help was positively related to family resources and the use of positive coping strategies.

Margalit and Yona (1991) compared the ability of family systems to cope (including perception of family climate and sense of coherence) in an Israeli kibbutz (49 families of nondisabled children and 43 families of disabled child) and in an Israeli city (48 families of disabled children, 51 families of non-disabled children). The results showed that parents of disabled children viewed their families as less supportive, as enabling less free expression of emotions, and as providing fewer opportunities for intellectual and recreational activities. Parent in the kibbutz environment reported fewer expressions of achievement orientation and fewer conflicts than did their city peers. The implication was that early designing the outcome study would be effective in promoting family strength. These gaps constitute the recommendations for future study direction in the area of the impact of factors on parental functioning.

Atkin's et al. (2000) study showed that parents of chronically ill child with sickle cell disease or thalassemia focused on their ability to manage and achieve mastery over the condition. The parents used normalization and positive framing to manage the condition. Information provision should increase locus of control and deal with the condition.

Silberberg (2001) used the triangular study with 605 families to find that self-identified strong families agreed with positive statements (e.g., strongly connected to each other, easy to share values and ideas, love one another, often laugh with each other, enjoying helping each other). She found eight qualities of family strength from 177 volunteers: communication, togetherness, commitment, sharing activities, affection, support, acceptance, and resilience. They also extracted two strength themes from 33 families: support from extended family and friends, and positive co-parenting arrangements. The major implication for nursing is a strengths-based approach that focuses on available resources and skills within the family and community, and the empowerment of the family and community in building resilience.

Influencing Factors Related to Family Function

Family hardiness, family support, and family communication

Based on the typology model of adjustment and adaptation, and the family stress model, Failla et al., (1991) addressed the interaction of key components that affect the functioning of families of children with developmental disability from 57 mothers. They predict satisfaction with family functioning. Results indicated positive relationships between family hardiness, coherence, and functional support, and satisfaction with family function. The major contribution is to note that family hardiness could diminish the effects of stress, increase the use of support, and facilitate adaptation. The sample size is too small to generalize or could use comparison group of families with normal children.

Olsen and colleagues (1999) studied 54 couples (108 parents) of young children with disabilities and found that income, family support, and incendiary communication predicted parent's hardiness; and family hardiness was positively related to family support for the mothers and fathers, but negatively related to define this incendiary communication. The major contribution is the assumption that families develop basic capabilities and strengths, which foster the development and growth of family members and protect them from major disruption during family changes or transitions. Health providers need to teach effective communication skills and conflict management, and to provide external sources of support. The sample size is enough and homogeneous in ethnicity and social status.

Family problem solving communication, family schema, and family meaning

McCubbin, & Thompson et al. (1998) gathered self-report data from 101 parents of Native Hawaiian preschool children. The result showed that family problem solving communication and family hardiness to be significant predictors to explain the variability in family dysfunction. Family schema is indirectly related to family dysfunction, primarily through coherence, hardiness, and family problem-solving communication. They also constructed a series of path models to account for indirect relationships of family schema and sense of coherence on levels of family functioning. A major strength of this study is the use of a conceptual framework as the basis of the study, and use of a randomly selected sample, thus making it a more reliable representation of the intended population of Native Hawaiian. But the limitation of the sample size and uniqueness induced limitation of the generalizability of the findings.

Cannors and Donnella's (1998) anthropological study was to explore parents' perception and coping abilities with eight Navajo families with autistic children and 24 other families without autism. Themes that emerged were concerned: cultural constructs of health and illness, child-rearing practices, and residential placement. Results showed that parents were concerned their children's competency, and residential placement. The implication for professionals is that family involve in the early childhood special education--family center approach, look at their own expectations and definitions of progress, provide a loving and caring relationship, and protection. The sample size is too small to generalize the cultural constructs.

Garwick, Kohrman, Titus, Wolman, and Blum (1999) designed a grounded theory method to interview 63 family caregivers of school children with chronic physical health impairments and used the Impact-on-Family Scale to discover how Hispanic, African-American, and European American families explain the cause of childhood chronic conditions and the indicators of resilience reflected in these explanations. The categories of explanation for the cause of childhood chronic conditions were: biomedical and environmental explanation; traditional and fatalistic beliefs; cause unknown; and personal attributions.

The major strength of the study is that the impact of traditional ethnocultural beliefs on families' explanations is most evident in descriptions of folk beliefs about illness and religious/spiritual interpretations of the chronic conditions. The influence of culture is also apparent in expressions of fatalistic and superstitious beliefs that reflect the family's worldview, thus contributing to theory refinement. A second area of strength is related to the development and refinement of psychometric measures of impact of attitudes and ethnic differences. The third major strength is the evidence of cumulative research in areas of family explanation's knowledge and attitudes toward minority patients and on the families' perceptions of cross-cultural health care behaviors. The primary limitation of this paper is that the sample size is too large for ground theory method, which is difficult to control the rigor, reliability, and validity, but too small for the quantitative design that is difficult to generalize and to compare the different beliefs in the three cluster groups. The important contribution of this research to date is the greater awareness and sensitivity that has emerged concerning cultural differences among the meaning the family attributes to the cause of the child's condition and which changes overtime.

Cohen et al. (2002) tried to use a qualitative ground theory method to explore fifteen Israeli women whose families underwent a crisis event. The authors found that family's abilities, system flexibility to shift roles, abilities of family members to give up their personal needs for someone else, and to accept other people's feeling promoted family resilience. Other contributive factors included a sense of humor, trust, and providing a sense of security. The implication of nursing practice was women's perception and definition of the resilience concept including expressiveness, self-disclosure, optimism, connectedness, flexibility, and family values in interpersonal relationship. Families should be encouraged to open and sincere in communication and intimate in personal relationships. The sample size was small and did not include males so the ability to generalize findings is limited. In addition, cultural diversity may influence the result of the perception of family resilience. The implication is that nursing intervention should focus on developing effective communication skills and conflict management, and provide external sources of support.

Family time together, life style, pile-up of stressors and strains

McCubbin (1998) used regression analysis with data gathered from 184 African American enlisted military personal and their spouses to determine factors most influential in helping them adjust to overseas assignments. The results revealed that military life style (coherence) and confidence in spouse's self-reliance, spouse employment, and spouse's assessment of family time together emerged as important factors associated with adaptation. The sampling of the study focused on African-American military families that reduced the generalizability of the finding to represent military or army families and their functioning. The strength of the research is four independent predictors can explain the variability in African-American enlisted family functioning to reassignment in Western Europe. The major contribution is that critical variables of the pile-up of stressors and strains, and particularly family strengths, supports, and coherence to be of central importance in explaining African-American enlisted family functioning.

Hawley (2000) based his study on the family resilience and narrative therapy model. He used longitudinal case study to understand family myths and family stories. The multiple major stressors were cancer, unemployment, financial insecurity, and marital separation. The major obstacle in the family was inability to communicate. Barriers to effective family relationships were finances, differences over religion, father's depression, and interference from mother's ex-husband. The therapy team helped the family discover resources to solve the problems, stabilize the family, bring the family to a higher level of functioning, and overcome the tremendous obstacles in holding their family together. The implication for clinical practice focused on family strengths and successes, developmental path, overcome obstacles to achieve well-being, and access outside resource. The weak point was the author never indicated the rigorous and saturation of the context about the narrative record.

Summary of Analysis and Critique of Research Literature Review

Among the reviewed articles, different research designs have been used to study family resiliency or related concepts (e.g., family coherence, family hardiness, family appraisal, family function, and family problem solving communication, and family adaptation). No articles combined both phases of the resiliency model. Most of them emphasized the adaptation phase. Researchers considered systems for maintaining rigor and promoting the continuity of family resilience; and more use of strengths-based approaches or resilience-based approaches to explore the concept. The attributes of the conceptual framework focused on family functioning that related to family's resilience. In other words, the family is ability to cope and restore family balance (Burr & Klein, 1994; Walsh, 1998).

Strengths

The major strengths of this set of studies are (a) family research has been stimulated in a wide variety of disciplines including epidemiology, sociology, psychology, psychiatry. The nursing professional must consider various variables including coherence, adaptation, hardiness, and resilience emerging in family therapy or designing social policy, nursing evaluation; and from more specialized areas related to substance abuse and delinquency; (b) identify a broad range of background conditions, personal characteristics, social relations and community resources that are essential to understanding healthy adaptation in the face of adversity; (c) explore the concept of resilience from multiple dimensional process of family resilience that include belief systems, organizational patterns, and communication processes, which were viewed as a functional units in the family; (d) Family resilience research has contributed to new ideas and insights in prevention and treatment programs. There is more of a focus on the family strength to facilitate skills and competence of family members.

Limitations

The limitations of these studies are (a) the use of a geographically limited sample. The majority of the studies were carried out in the Native American, immigrant, and African-American families; (b) none of the study included families with a genetic disease such as DMD; (c) only one utilized an adequate sample of parents of young children with a disability; (d) only one used the anthropology design method to explore cultural resilience and the sample was limited to Navajo families; (e) no repeated testing and refinement of the resilience model of family stress, adjustment, and adaptation scale; (f) in most studies the sample size was too small to generalize the body of resilience knowledge.

Gaps

There has been little research directly to focus on family resilience of children with disabilities. Early studies reported more stress of families with mental disability most focused on the adult. Among the review articles, it is difficult to find articles that explore the following views:(a) making meaning of adversity, illness, or disability; (b) focus on the positive outlook in the face of the adversity, learning optimism and finding humor, sustain hope; (c) health professional belief: treatment and healing, badly strained relationship may remain unhealed; and (d) future expectation and fear of the families. Individual concepts have been developed for family hardiness, family of coherence, family function, family schema, family resources, and family appraisal. However, different research designs and different measurements induced different models. So the resiliency model could continue to develop in the nursing area. Use of one family member as an informant in family resilience research is a biased perspective of family phenomena. It is suggested to measure the responses of multiple family members to gain greater perception into family phenomena. Researchers have some limitations in the resilience model because no article combines both instruments of adjustment and adaptation, and a few articles uses path analysis to check the model. Even though there were some articles presented from a nursing situation, most of them addressed some concepts from the resilience model that were not complete because they were concerned with the cultural diversity or the ability of human concentration.

Implication

The knowledge of the resilience model can be useful in designing family-based prevention or treatment programs. Ethnic and culture backgrounds are critical elements in family adaptation and in the appraisal and relational processes families use to manage change and adaptation. It is necessary, therefore, for nursing professionals to understand the process and experience of families undergoing family changes or family crisis in order to facilitate their adaptation. Clinical implications include: (a) define the normal family influence, the standard by which families are judged on being normal and healthy. (b) develop caregiver education and support. (c) policy implication for more effective support and management of chronic illness in the home is worth looking at. Professionals can explore family support, family communication, and family hardiness in a family with a child with disability to help families develop insights and behaviors associated with hardiness. They also can teach effective communication skills and conflict management, and provide external sources of support.

Family resilience research in nursing implication is (a) to develop a mode of help to minimize threats to family integrity and facilitate healthy adaptation to caring for a child with special needs, and meet the challenges of change; (b) to examine the role of competency-enhancing help in adaptation process for mothers of children with special needs; (c) to assess impact of family factors on psychological morbidity of the mothers and relatives of a person with schizophrenia; (d) to determine the relationship between family coping and resources and family adjustment and parental stress in acute phase; (e) to examine relationships among family demands, family resources, family problem-solving communication, family coping and sibling well-being in families with disability; and finds (g) family resources play an important role in family adaptation to the ongoing challenges associated with raising a child with a chronic condition; (f) family with an affirming style of problem-solving communication adapt more successfully to stressful situations than families with an incendiary style of problem-solving communication.

Future Study

In the future, therefore, a longitudinal study would help to examine the process of family resilience in other diseases and life events. In addition, gender and cultural diversity may influence the outcome of the family resilience process. Research is not only concerned with both variables but it also has to consider family relationships, family resources, family communication, adaptation, and social support network. To identify cultural and social diversity in family resilience, qualitative research must focus on the family schema and family appraisal to organize both adjustment and adaptation, and designing intervention programs to increase family resources must also be considered.

What is the family crisis meaning?

Family crisis is a period of family disorganization, family disharmony, and imbalance in the system, which moves to the onset of the adaptation phase. Family crisis means the family is becoming unstable, disorganized, and dysfunctional. When families emerged in crisis, experienced disharmony, imbalance, and deterioration in the face of risk factors, they have their own recovery factors, capacities, and resources to change their patterns of functioning and to facilitate their adaptation. The recovery factors include family support, problem solving coping skills, family optimism and mastery, family advocacy, family meaning, and family schema (McCubbin et al., 1997). Families in crisis can transform danger into opportunity and challenge.

What is family vulnerability?

Family vulnerability means the family system deteriorated and is dysfunctional. When families are vulnerable, protective factors fashion the family's ability to stand risk factors and to adjust. The protective factors include family hardiness, family communication, financial management, support network, family bonding, and family time (Family resiliency, 2002).

Both risk and recovery factors are the predictable variables of the resilience model. The family with a disabled child will get more information to adapt to the multi-factors in the long-term life of the disability if researchers can explore all the factors of family resilience and provide the program for strengthening family function. Families in crisis can transform danger into opportunity and challenge.

What's Importance of Noting Family Resilience?

The human being and nature are interrelated and independent. The child with a physical or medical disability has an effect on each the other family members and on the family unit itself (Lynch & Morley, 1995). Therefore, to understand the importance of resilience in a family with a disabled child, we must acknowledge the cultural diversity and socioeconomic disparity of the family unit, as well as the core concept of disability policy.

Without understanding the culture and belief systems of the family and the phenomena of the relationship and communicational processes between the individual and the family, nursing could not be a holistic science. Changes affecting the family unit, such as the nuclear family structure, limited resource, racial discrimination, and economic upheaval have increased stress and decreased support and family adaptation.

Studies have assessed families as units rather than collections of perceptions from individual family members. McCubbin, Balling, Possin, Frierdich, and Bryne (2002) identify family resilience factors from parents of children with leukemia; and Thompson (1999) indicated the significance and meaning of an AIDS diagnosis and progression from mothers and adult children. There are a lot of methods to collect data from more than one family member, and then deal with these reports into something that is supposed to represent the family.

Especially, state government has invested a lot of budget to support disability groups (Beach Center on Families and Disability, 2002). Researchers analyze 110 policy leader respondents and identify eighteen core concepts of disability policy: anti-discrimination, autonomy, empowerment and participatory decision-making, privacy and confidentiality, liberty, protection from harm, cultural responsiveness, accountability, family integrity and unity, family centeredness, service coordination and collaboration, prevention, system capacity development, individualized and appropriate services, capacity based services, classification, productivity and contribution, and integration (Beach Center on Families and Disability, 2002). All the terminologies of the concept are similar to resilience characteristics and social resource or family resilience. Resilience applied to family helps families to resist to disruption in the face of change and adapt in the face of the crisis, offers families an opportunity to change in constructive ways and to strengthen family bonds. Nursing professionals have to approach the experiences of family resilience for the family with a disabled child. Nursing professionals have to approach the experiences of family resilience for the family with a disabled child.

References

Adrian, S. (2002). Disability defined. *Psychology Today, 35*, 34.

Antonovsky, A., & Sourani, T. (1988). Family sense of coherence. *Journal of Marriage and the Family, 50*, 79-92.

Atkin, K., & Ahmad, W. I. U. (2000). Family care-giving and chronic illness: How parents cope with a child a sickle cell disorder or thalassaemia. *Health and Social Care in the Community, 8*, 57-69.

Beach Center on Families and Disability. (2002). *Core concepts of disability policy. University of Kansas.* University of Kansas. Retrieved June 2002, 2002, from the World Wide Web: http://www.beachcenter.org/main.pp3?page_id=2

Benard, B. (2001). *Fostering resiliency in kids: Protective factors in the family, school, and community.* Western Regional Center for Drug-free School and Community. San Francisco. Retrieved April 5, 2002, from the World Wide Web: http://www.divorceandkids.com/Parent20Tips/resiliency.htm

Bennett, T., & DeLuca, D. A. (1996). Families of children with disabilities: Positive adaptation across the life cycle. *Social Work in Education, 18*, 31-44.

Braverman, M. T. (2001). *Family resiliency: Building strengths to meet life's changes.* Focus: Spring.

Bristor, M. M. (1991). The birth of a handicapped child: A wholistic model for grieving. In R. P. Marinelli & A. E. Dell Orto (Eds.), *The psychological and social impact of disability* (pp. 59-80). New York: Springer.

Brown, L. (1993). *The new shorter Oxford English Dictionary on historical principles* (Vol. 2). Oxford: Clarendon.

Burr, W. R., & Klein, S. R. (1994). *Reexamining family stress.* Thousand Oaks, CA: Sage.

Cannors, J. L., & Donnellan, A. M. (1998). Walk in Beauty: Western Perspectives on disability and Navajo Family/Cultural resilience. In H. I. McCubbin & E. A. Thompson & A. I. Thompson & J. E. Fromer (Eds.), *Resiliency in Native America and Immigrant Families* (pp. 159-182). Thousand Oaks, CA: Sage.

Cohen, O., Slonim, I., Finzi, R., & Leichtentritt, R. D. (2002). Family resilience: Israeli mothers' perspectives. *American Journal of Family Therapy, 30*, 173-187.

Dyson, L. L. (1997). Fathers and mothers of school-age children with developmental disabilities: Parental stress, family functioning, and social support. *American Journal on Mental Retardation, 102,* 267-279.

Epstein, N., Baldwin, L., & Bishop, D. (1983). The McMaster family assessment device. *Journal of Marital and Family Therapy, 9,* 17 l- 180.

Failla, S., & Jones, L. C. (1991). Families of children with developmental disabilities: An examination of family hardiness. *Research in Nursing & health, 14,* 41-50.

Family resiliency. (2002). Retrieved August 11, 2002, from the World Wide Web: http://www.extension.iastate.edu/families/Resiliency/qa.html

Flexner, S. B., & Hauck, L. C. (1993). *Random house unabridged dictionary.* New York: Random house.

Garwick, A. W., Kohrman, C. H., Titus, J. C., Wolman, C., & Blum, R. W. (1999). Variations in families' explanations of childhood chronic conditions: A cross cultural perspective. In H. I. McCubbin & E. A. Thompson & A. I. Thompson & J. A. Futrell (Eds.), *The dynamics of resilient families* (pp. 165-202). Thousand Oaks, CA: Sage.

Gottlieb, A. (1998). Single mother of children with disabilities: the role of sense of coherence in managing multiple challenges. In J. E. Fromer (Ed.), *Stress, coping, and health in families: sense of coherence and resilience* (pp. 189-206). Thousand Oaks, CA: Sage.

Hawley, D., & De Haan, L. (1996). Towards a definition of family resilience: Integrating individual and family perspectives. *Family Process, 35,* 283-298.

Hawley, D. R. (2000). Clinical implications of family resilience. *American Journal of Family Therapy, 28,* 101-126.

Hill, R. (1949). *Families under stress.* New York: Harper & Row.

Hill, R. (1958). Generic features of families under stress. *Social Casework, 49,* 139-150.

Institue for Health and Disability. (1997). A new way to think about cultural sensitivity: Families share their understanding of disabilities. *Health Issues for Children & Youth and their family, 5*(1), 1-12.

Judge, S. L. (1998). Parental coping strategies and strengths in families of young childen with disabilities. *Family Relations, 47,* 262-267.

Kazak, A. E. (1992). The social context of coping with childhood chronic illness: Family systems and social support. In A. M. La Greca & L. J. Siegel & J. L. Wallander & C. E. Walker (Eds.), *Stress and coping in child health* (pp. 262-278). New York: Guilford.

Knussen, C., & Sloper, P. (1992). Stress in families of children with disability: A review of risk and resistance factors. *Journal of Mental Health, 1*, 241-256.

Kosciulek, J. F., McCubbin, M. A., & McCubbin, H. I. (1993). A theoretical framework for family adaptation to head injury. *Journal of Rehabilitation, 59*, 40-45.

Lustig, D. (1997). Families with an adult with mental retardation: empirical family typologies. *Rehabilitation Counseling Bulletin, 41*, 138-157.

Luthar, S. S., Cicchetti, D., & Beck, B. (2000). The construct of resilience: A critical evaluation and guidelines for future work. *Child Development, 71*, 543-562.

Lynch, R. T., & Morley, K. L. (1995). Adaptation to pediatric physical disability with the family system: A conceptual model for counseling families. *Family Journal, 3*, 207-216.

Margalit, M., & Yona, L. (1991). Community support in Israeli kibbutz and city families of children with disabilities: Family climate and parental coherence. *Journal of Special Education, 24*, 427-440.

McCubbin, H. I. (1998). Resiliency in African American families: Military families in foreign environments. In H. I. McCubbin & E. A. Thompson & A. I. Thompson & J. A. Futrell (Eds.), *Resiliency in African-American families*. Thousand Oaks, CA: Sage.

McCubbin, H. I., Balling, K., Possin, P., Frierdich, S., & Bryne, B. (2002). Family resiliency in childhood cancer. *Family Relations, 51*, 103-111.

McCubbin, H. I., & McCubbin, M. A. (1988). Typologies of resilient families: Emerging roles of social class and ethnicity. *Family Relations, 37*, 247-254.

McCubbin, H. I., McCubbin, M. A., & Thompson, A. I. (1993). Resiliency in families: The role of family schema and appraisal in family adaptation to Crises. In T. H. Brubaker (Ed.), *Family relations: Challenge for the future* (Vol. I, pp. 153-177). Newbury Park, CA: Sage.

McCubbin, H. I., McCubbin, M. A., Thompson, A. I., Han, S. Y., & Allen, C. T. (1997). *Families under stress: What makes them resilient*. 1997 AAFCS Commemorative Lecture. Retrieved August 8, 2002, from the World Wide Web: http://www.cyfernet.extension.umn.edu/research/resilient.html

McCubbin, H. I., McCubbin, M. A., Thompson, A. I., & Thompson, E. I. (1998). Resiliency in ethic families: A conceptual model for predicting family adjustment and adaptation.

In J. E. Fromer (Ed.), *Resiliency in Native American and immigrant families* (pp. 3-48). Thousand Oaks, CA: Sage.

McCubbin, H. I., & Patterson, J. M. (1981). *Systematic assessment of family stress, resource, and coping: Tools for research, education, and clinical intervention*. St. Paul, MN: Department of Family Social Science.

McCubbin, H. I., & Patterson, J. M. (1983). The family stress process: The Double ABCX Model of adjustment and adaptation. In H. I. McCubbin & M. Sussman & J. M. Patterson (Eds.), *Advances and development in family stress theory and research* (pp. 7-37). New York: Haworth.

McCubbin, H. I., Thompson, A. I., Elver, K. E., & Carpenter, K. (1992). *The family (ethnicity) schema index*. Madison, WI: University of Wisconsin, Family Stress, Coping, & Health Project.

McCubbin, H. I., Thompson, A. I., & McCubbin, M. A. (1996). *Family assessment: Resiliency, coping and adaptation: Inventories for research and practice*. Madison, WI: University of Wisconsin Publisher.

McCubbin, H. I., Thompson, A. I., Thompson, E. A., Elver, K. M., & McCubbin, M. A. (1998). Ethnicity, schema, and coherence: Appraisal processes for families in crisis. In J. E. Fromer (Ed.), *Stress, coping, and health in families: Sense of coherence and resiliency* (pp. 41-67). Madison, WI: University of Wisconsin Press.

McCubbin, M. A. (1993). Family stress theory and the development of nursing knowledge about family adaptation. In S. L. Feetham & S. B. Meister & J. M. Beil & C. L. Gillis (Eds.), *The nursing of families: Theory, research, education, and practice* (pp. 46-58). Newbury Park, CA: Sage.

McCubbin, M. A., & McCubbin, H. I. (1987). Family stress theory and assessment: The T-Double ABCX model of family adjustment and adaptation. In H. I. McCubbin & A. I. Thompson (Eds.), *Family assessment inventories for research and practice* (pp. 3-32). Madison, WI: University of Wisconsin-Madison.

McCubbin, M. A., & McCubbin, H. I. (1993). Family coping with health crises: the resiliency model of family stress, adjustment and adaptation. In C. Danielson & B. Hamel-Bissell & P. Winstead-Fry (Eds.), *Families, Health and Illness: Perspectives on coping and intervention* (pp. 21-63). St. Louis: Mosby.

McIntyre, C. L. (2000). *The role of competency-enhancing helpgiving practice in parental adaptation for families of children with special needs.* Unpublished Ph. D Dissertation, University of Texas at Austin, Austin, Texas.

Olsen, S. F. O., Marshall, E. S., Mandleco, B. L., Allred, K. W., Dyches, T. T., & Sansom, N. (1999). Supporting, communication, and hardiness in families with children with disabilities. *Journal of Family Nursing, 5,* 275-291.

Olson, D., Portner, J., & Bell, R. (1982). *FACES II: Family adaptability and cohesion evaluation scales.* St. Paul, MN: Family Social Science, University of Minnesota.

Olson, D., Sprenkle, D., & Russell, C. (1979). Circumplex model of marital and family systems: I. Cohesion and adaptability dimensions, family types and clinical applications. *Family Process, 18,* 3-28.

Patterson, J. M. (1988). Family experiencing stress: I. The family adjustment and adaptation response model, II. Applying the FAAR model to health-related issues for intervention and research. *Family System Medicine, 6,* 202-237.

Patterson, J. M. (2002). *Promoting resilience in families experiencing stress.* University of Minnesota, School of Public Health. Retrieved August 6, 2002, from the World Wide Web: http://www..epi.umi.edu/epi_pages/Syllabi/reading2.html

Patterson, J. M., & McCubbin, H. I. (1983). Chronic illness: Family stress and coping. In H. I. McCubbin (Ed.), *Stress and the family: Volume II: Coping with Catastrophe* (pp. 21-36). New York: Brunner/Mazel.

Robison, N., & Davidson, G. (1996). *Chambers 21st Century Dictionary.* England: Chamber.

Silberberg, S. (2001). Searching for family resilience. *Family Matters, 58,* 52-61.

Silliman, B., & Pike, L. B. (2002). *Family resiliency factors commonly identified in research.* In 1994 Resiliency research review: Conceptual & research foundations. Retrieved February 15, 2002, from the World Wide Web: http://www.cyfernet.org/research/resilreview.htm

Simmerman, S., & Blacher, J. (2001). Fathers' and mothers' perceptions of father involvement in families with young children with a disability. *Journal of Intellectual & Developmental Disability, 26,* 325-338.

Tak, Y. R., & McCubbin, M. (2002). Family stress, perceived social support and coping following the diagnosis of a child's congenital heart disease. *Journal of Advanced Nursing, 39,* 190-198.

Thames, B., & Thomason, D. J. (2000). *Building family strengths resiliency. Clemson Extension: Family Relationships.* Retrieved, from the World Wide Web: http://virtual.clemson.edu/groups/psapublishing/Pages/FYD/FL529.pdf

Thompson, E. A. (1999). Resiliency in families with a member facing AIDS. In E. A. McCubbin & E. A. Thompson & A. I. Thompson & J. A. Futrell (Eds.), *The dynamics of resilient families* (pp. 135-164). Thousand Oaks, CA: Sage.

Thompson, E. A., McCubbin, H. I., Thompson, A. I., & Elver, K. M. (1998). Vulnerability and resiliency in native Hawaiian families under stress. In H. I. McCubbin & E. A. Thompson & A. I. Thompson & J. E. Fromer (Eds.), *Resiliency in native American and immigrant families* (pp. 115-132). Thousand Oaks, CA: Sage.

Walsh, F. (1998). *Strengthening family resilience.* New York: Guilford Press.

Walsh, F. (2002). A family resilience framework: innovative practice application. *Family Relations, 51,* 130-137.

Wisensale, S. K. (1993). State and federal initiatives in family policy. In T. H. Brubaker (Ed.), *Family relations: Challenges for the future* (Vol. 1, pp. 229-250). Newbury Park, CA: Sage.

Wolin, S. J., & Wolin, S. (1993). *The resilient self: how survivors of troubled families rise above adversity.* New York: Villard.

Part Three

Logical Inquiry through the Research Process

What Do Research Connect to Go?

The resilience model has been studied with a number of families dealing with chronic illness, disability, adversity, and trauma. The criteria of review articles selected was based on the subject coming from a family with a disabled child, or selected because measurements were with the whole family resilience model but with a non-disabled family. The researcher depended on the relationship of predictor variables of family resiliency model to analyze and critique. Related factors of family adaptation were first analyzed. Then related factors of family function were described.

After reviewing the articles, we know there are 4 factors that influence family adaptation: sense of coherence and using of resource, stress related to emotional climate and pessimism concerning the child future, social support and family strengths; and there are 3 factors that influence family function: family hardiness, family support, and family communication; family problem solving communication, family schema, and family meaning; family time together, life-style, pile-up of stressors and strains. The following discusses these factors.

Among the reviewed articles, different research designs have been used to study family resiliency or related concept (e.g., family coherence, family hardiness, family appraisal, family function, and family problem solving communication, and family adaptation). No articles combing both of two phases of the resiliency model. Most of them emphasized adaptation phase. Researchers considered system ways to maintain rigor and promote the continuity of family resiliency; and more use of strengths-based approaches or resilience-based approaches to explore the concept, conceptual framework attribute focused on family functioning that related to family resilience the family ability to cope and restore family balance (Walsh, 1998).

Strengths

The major strengths of this set of studies are (a) family research has stimulated research in a wide variety of disciplines including epidemiology, sociology, psychology, psychiatry, and nursing professional to consider various variables including coherence, adaptation, hardiness, and resilience emerging in family therapy or designing social policy, nursing evaluation; and from more specialized areas related to substance to delinquency; (b) identity a broad range of background conditions, personals characteristic, social relations and community resources that are essential to understanding healthy adaptation in face the adversity; (c) explore concept of resilience from multiple dimensional process of family resilience that included belief system, organizational patterns, and communication processes, which were viewed as a functional units in the family; (d) Family resiliency research has contributed to new ideas and insights in prevention and treatment programs. There is more of a focus on the family strength to facilitate skills and competence of family members.

Limitations

The limitations of these studies are (a) the use of a geographically limited sample. The majority of the studies were carried out in the Native American, immigrant, and African-American families; (b) none of the study included genetic disease families with physical disability such as DMD in the sample; (c) only one utilized an adequate sample of parents of young children with disability; (d) only one used of the anthropology design method to explore cultural resilience and sample limited at Navajo family; (e) no repeated testing and refinement of resilience model of family stress, adjustment, and adaptation scale; (f) most studies the sample size was too small to generalize the body of resilience knowledge.

What kind of implication of study finding?

The knowledge of the resiliency model can be useful in designing family-based prevention or treatment programs. Ethical and culture is critical elements in family adaptation and in the appraisal and relational processes families use to manage change and adaptation. It is necessary, therefore, for nursing professionals to understand the process and experience of families undergoing family changes or family crisis in order to be facilitate their adaptation. Clinical implications include: (a) define the normal family influence the standard by which families are judging emphasis on being normal and health. (b) develop caregiver education and support. (c) policy implication for more effective support and management of chronic illness in the home is worth to concern. Professionals can explore family support, family communication, and family hardiness in family with a child with disabilities to help families develop insights and behaviors associated with hardiness, teach effective communication skills and conflict management, and provide external sources of support.

Family resiliency research in nursing implication try (a) to develop mode of help to minimize threats to family integrity and facilitate healthy adaptation to caring for a child with special needs, and meet the challenges of change; (b) to examine the role of competency-enhancing help in adaptation process for mothers of children with special needs; (c) to assess impact of family factors on psychological morbidity of the mothers and relatives of a person with schizophrenia; (d) to determine the relationship between family coping and resources and family adjustment and parental stress in acute phase; (e) to examine relationship among family demands, family resources, family problem-solving communication, family coping and sibling well-being in families with disability; and finds (g) family resources play an important role in family adaptation to the ongoing challenge associated with raising a child with a chronic condition; (f) family with an affirming style of problem-solving communication adapt more successfully to stressful situations than families with an incendiary style of problem-solving communication.

What gaps are in the literature review?

Among the review articles, it is difficult to find articles to explore the follows views:(a) the making meaning of adversity, illness, or disability; (b) focus on the positive outlook in the face of the adversity, learning optimism and finding humor, sustain hope; (c) health professional belief: treatment and healing, badly strained relationship may remain unhealed; and (d) future expectation and fear of the families. Family hardiness, family of coherence, family function, family schema, family resources, and family appraisal have been developed their individual concept. However, different research designs and different measurements induced different model. So the resiliency model could continue to develop in the nursing area.

Use of one family member as an informant in family resiliency research is a biased perspective of family phenomena. It has to suggest measuring the responses of multiple family members to gain greater perception into family phenomena. There was the limitation to insight the resiliency model because no article combining both instruments of adjustment and adaptation, and no article use path analysis to check the model. Even though there were some articles presented from nursing situation, most of them dressed some of concepts from the resiliency model that were not complete because they concern the culture diversity, or ability of human concentration.

Where do we need to go next?

In the future, therefore, extending to any kind of pattern of disease or life events of stress and longitudinal work to examine the process of family resilience. In addition, gender and cultural diversity may influence the outcome of family resilience process. Research not only concerns both variables but also has to consider family relationships, family resources, family communication, adaptation, and social support network. Family schema and family appraisal need to consider the cultural and social diversity to do the qualitative research to organize both of adjustment and adaptation, and design the intervention program to increase family resources would be considered.

What are Changes in Society Affecting Family Ability to Cope?

The philosophical and policy trends of de-institutionalization and normalization encourage families to raise children with developmental disabilities at home. Advances in medical science and changes in public policy have resulted in more disabled children supported in the community and at home. Political, economic, and demographic changes have complicated the family policy as society evolves into a multiracial, multicultural, and multilingual society. Four important trends in a socio-historical context are: "diverse family forms," "changing gender roles and relations," "cultural diversity and socioeconomic disparity," and "varying and expanded family life cycle course".

What are Key Components in Evaluation of Family Resilience Research?

There are five key components to evaluate: (a) family stressors and family strains; (b) family resources; (c) family problem solving and coping; (d) family appraisal, family coherence, and family schema; and (e) family adaptation.

What are the major concepts of the family resilience?

McCubbin, Thompson, and McCubbin (1996) defined **family stressor** as a demand placed on the family that produces changes in the family system. The stressor may threaten the stability of the family units or place significant demands on the family's resources and capabilities.

Family resource is a family's capabilities and strengths to resist a crisis and promote family resilience to establish patterns of function and achieve harmony and balance. The characteristic of hardiness is a stress resistance and adaptation resource that refers to the internal strengths and durability of the family unit.

Family problem solving and coping indicate the action that reflect a family's ability to deal with the stressor and hardship to maintain or restore the family harmony and balance.

Family appraisal is the family perception of the seriousness of a disability and its hardships. It contains family beliefs and expectations regarding disability. It was defined as a familial sense of coherence. It was measured using the Family Sense of Coherence.

Family schema is a structure of fundamental convictions, values, beliefs, and expectations (McCubbin et al., 1996; McCubbin, Thompson, Thompson, Elver, & McCubbin, 1998). A family schema includes cultural-ethical beliefs, and values. It was measured using the Family (Ethnicity) Schema Index (McCubbin, Thompson et al., 1998).

Family cohesion is defined as the emotional bonding among family members and the degree of personal autonomy experienced in the family, as well as the degree of family adaptability (Olson, Sprenkle, & Russell, 1979). **Family adaptability** is defined as the ability of the family system to change its power structure, roles, and rules in response to situational and developmental stress (McCubbin et al., 1996). It was measured using the Family Adaptability and Cohesion Evaluation Scale (Olson, Portner, & Bell, 1982).

Family adaptation is the outcome of the family's efforts in response to family stressors and is defined as a minimal discrepancy between demands and capabilities (McCubbin et al., 1996), and to bring a new or satisfactory level of balance, harmony, coherence, and functioning to family crisis situations (McCubbin et al., 1996). It was measured using the Family Assessment Device (Epstein, Baldwin, & Bishop, 1983).

Review the articles what influencing factors related to family adaptation?

There are 4 factors that influence family adaptation: sense of coherence and using of resource, stress related to emotional climate and pessimism concerning the child future, social support, and family strengths.

Review the articles what influencing factors related to family adaptation?

There are 3 group of factors that influence family functioning: family hardiness, family support, and family communication; family problem solving communication, family schema, and family meaning; family time together, life-style, pile-up of stressors and strains.

What's the big factor and quality for the physical disabled children?

Depend to a large degree on the parents' ability to love the child completely. In addition, socio-economic or material resource, locus of control, self-esteem, relationship with the family and social network, and service response can provide resistance against stress.

What are the results of current researches?

Use of social support was highly associated with family strengths (Judge, 1998). Dyson (1997) found that although fathers and mothers of children with disabilities did not differ in levels of parental stress, social support, or family functioning; parental stress was related to family problems due to the child's special needs, to the family's emotional climate, and to parents' pessimism concerning the child's future.

Lustig (1997) studied 116 parents of adult children with mental retardation. Results indicated that most families were resilient and functioning positive. There were positive correlations between scores on family adaptation, and social support, family sense of coherence, and family adaptability

Single mothers' sense of coherence was associated with family coherence. They had a strong sense of coherence and greater use of resources then they had more adaptive outcomes (Gottlieb, 1998). Kazak (1992) indicated that the quality and nature of the family environment and the quantity and efficacy of informal support systems utilized by families helped to explain variation in parental and family adaptation to a typical parenting experience.

Appropriate professional support helps to reduce stress and facilitate coping by offering information, financial, help and emotional support. Health providers can empower families to care for their disabled children by coordinate various medical care, making care accessible, and providing an appropriate service delivery system (Atkin and Ahmad, 2000—Thalassemia, & sickle cell).

Use of networks disabled child's parents got (a) emotional support and caregiving from families and friends; (b) emotional outlet and source of information from parent groups; (c) development of ideas and actions and support from professionals (Bennett and Deluca, 1996). Parents of disabled children viewed their families as less supportive, as enabling less free expression of emotions, and as providing fewer opportunities for intellectual and recreational activities (Margalit and Yona, 1991). There is positive relationship between family hardiness, coherence, and functional support, and satisfaction with family function.

Olsen and colleagues (1999) studied 54 couples (108 parents) of young children with disabilities and found that income, family support, and incendiary communication predicted parent's hardiness; and family hardiness was positively related to family support for the mothers and fathers, but negatively related to define this incendiary communication.

Family problem solving communication and family hardiness are significant predictors to explain the variability in family dysfunction. Family schema is indirectly related to family dysfunction, primarily through coherence, hardiness, and family problem-solving communication.

What are implications of the current researches?

Appropriate professional support helps to reduce stress and facilitate coping by offering information, financial, help and emotional support. Health providers can empower families to care for their disabled children by coordinate various medical care, making care accessible, and providing an appropriate service delivery system. A social network has an effect on family adaptation. Professional needs to know how to inquire about family schema and recognize importance of family appraisal in shaping family function, adjustment, and adaptation. Early designing the outcome study would be effective in promoting family strength. Family hardiness could diminish the effects of stress, increase the use of support, and facilitate adaptation. Women's perception and definition of the resilience concept included expressiveness, self-disclosure, optimism, connectedness, flexibility, and family values in interpersonal relationship. Families should be encouraged to open and sincere in communication and intimate in personal relationships.

Part Four

Review of Theory and Measurement

Theory and Measurement of the Family Resilience Construct

Introduction

A family resilience approach intends to identify and reinforce interactional processes that enable families to resist and rebound from disruptive life challenges (Walsh, 1998). In order to support and strengthen families with a disabled child, we need to use conceptual tools to approach clinical intervention, prevention efforts, research, and family policy. Disability means an incapacity or disqualification from normal life. A child with a disability means the child is deprived of physical and/or mental abilities. Disabling conditions are life-long and often require services from many agencies that increase financial costs, caregiver burdens, and social isolation, as well as restricting life-styles and career opportunities (Failla & Jones, 1991; Gottlieb, 1998; Patterson & McCubbin, 1983). In past decades, much of existing research has focused on negative indicators of response (e.g., depression, anxiety), rather than positive indicators (competence, self-esteem). A family resilience framework fundamentally alters traditional deficit-based approaches to research and practice.

Purpose of the Paper

The purpose of this paper is to describe: (a) overviews of the literature on the theoretical background of family resilience, its determinants and consequences and the way family resilience is supposed to be measured in general; (b) an operationalization of the measurement of family resilience when applied to the psycho-socio domain of families of children with disabilities.

Defining Resilience

Resilience in an individual refers to successful adaptation despite risk and adversity (Masten, 1994). Resilience is derived from the individual's perception and experience. Resilience is a manifestation of competence despite exposure to significant stressors. Examining definitions of resilience in dictionaries and articles, most authors used the terms "ability", "power", or "capacity" to recover, overcome, resist, or bounce back from misfortune and adversity (Walsh, 2002). Some used "change", "resist", or "cultivate strengths" to positively meet the challenge of life (Brown, 1993; Flexner & Hauck, 1993; Robinson & Davidson, 1996). Walsh (1998) defined resilience as "the capacity to rebound from adversity strengthened and more resourceful" (p.4). The Chinese word of "crisis" has two meanings, "danger" and "opportunity", to change and improve (Walsh, 1998). Resilience is "forged through adversity" (p.6). Resilience is a concept that incorporates two components: (a) exposure to significant stressors or risks, and (b) demonstration of competence and successful adaptation (Braverman, 2001).

Defining Family Resilience

The term "family resilience" refers to coping and adaptational processes in the family as a functional unit. Family processes mediate stress and enable families to surmount crisis and weather prolonged hardship (Braverman, 2001, p.14). Family resilience is the family's ability to exhibit strengths to positively face the challenge of life. The primary variables associated with resilience in families, including commitment, communication, cohesion, adaptability, spirituality, time together, connectedness, and efficacy (Silliman & Pike, 2002). Hawley and De Haan (1996) indicated that family resilience represented adaptive path in the face of stress. Resilient families can positively respond to the interactive combination of risk and recovery factors, and share beliefs or feelings (Hawley & De Haan, 1996). The emerging Institute for Health and Disability (1997), Walsh (1998), Cohen et al. (2002), and Silliman and Pike (2002) have discussed how resilient families with a child with a chronic condition can balance the demands of each other in the family; maintain social integration, a positive outlook, commitment, family boundaries, flexibility, time together, and connectedness; and develop communication competence and open emotional expression; to collaborate relationships with professionals (collaborative problem solving); and make meaning of adversity and the flexibility to shift roles and provide support.

Sources of Family Resilience

Family resilience beliefs are influenced by two important sources of phases: vulnerability VS adjustment and crisis VS adaptation. Vulnerability is the most important source of family resilience because it is based on a person's or families own experience. McCubbin and Paterson (1983) defined "adjustment as a short-term response that is characterized by first-order change" (p. 25). They proposed that adjustment is most relevant as a response to normative change, and adaptation is a response to nonnormative change (McCubbin & McCubbin, 1988). Adjustment involves the minimal transitory changes to face the risk factors; the influence recovery factors will facilitate the family's ability and efforts to maintain its integrity, functioning, and fulfill developmental tasks. Adaptation involves the function of recovery factors that promote the family's ability to "bounce back" and adapt in family crisis situations (McCubbin, McCubbin et al., 1998).

Once a family has high resilience, they tend to generalize a belief system, organize process, and communication (Walsh, 1998). The effects of failure depend on the family function, family resource, family schema, family hardiness, and problem solving skills. In illness situations, especially chronic illness or disability, however, hardships are often numerous and severe, demanding more changes in the family system, and the family may experience maladjustment and a resulting state of crisis. Family crisis is a period of family disorganization, family disharmony, and imbalance in the system, which moves to the onset of the adaptation phase.

Operational Definitions of Key Components Are Discussed Under

Major Components of the Concept Framework

Depending on nursing process to explore resilience in family with a disabled child, there are five key components to evaluate: (a) family stressors and family strains; (b) family resources; (c) family problem solving and coping; (d) family appraisal, family coherence, and family schema; (e) family adaptation.

Family stressors

McCubbin, Thompson, and McCubbin (1996) defined family stressor as a demand placed on the family that produces changes in the family system (e.g., life cycle, family boundary, family type). The stressor may threaten the stability of the family units or places significant demands on the family's resources and capabilities. A family type is a set of attributes that produce predictable and discernible patterns of family functioning (McCCubin et al., 1996).

Family resources

The term was described as a family's capabilities and strengths to resist a crisis and promote family resilience to establish patterns of function and achieve harmony and balance (McCubbin et al., 1996). Hardiness contains three components: control, commitment, and challenge. Family hardiness specifically refers to the internal strengths and durability of the family unit, a sense of control over the outcomes of life events and hardships, a view of change as beneficial and growth producing, an active orientation in adjusting to and managing stressful situations (McCubbin, et al., 1996). Family hardiness focused on family patterned approach to life's hardships and its' typical pattern of appraising the impact of life events and changes on family functioning.

Family problem solving and coping

These terms indicate as the action that family's ability to deal with the stressor and hardship to maintain or restore the family harmony and balance. Adaptive coping strategies and problem solving communication patterns are more generalized ways of responding to family hardship and difficulties by creating a family environment.

Family appraisal, family coherence, and family schema

Family appraisal is the family perception of the seriousness of a disability and its hardships. It contains family beliefs and expectations regarding disability. It was defined as a familial sense of coherence. Family schema is a structure of fundamental conviction, values, beliefs, and expectations (McCubbin, Thompson, & McCubbin, 1996; McCubbin, Thompson, Thompson, Elver, & McCubbin, 1998). A family schema includes cultural, ethical beliefs, and values. It is a generalized structure of shared values, beliefs, goals, expectations and priorities, shaped and adopted by the family unit, thus formulating a generalized informational structure against and through which information and experiences are compared, shifted, and processed. Family cohesion is defined as the emotional bonding among family members and the degree of personal autonomy experienced in the family, as well as the degree of family adaptability, defined as the ability of the family system to change its power structure, roles, and rules in response to situational and developmental stress.

Family adaptation

Family adaptation is the outcome of the family's efforts in response to family stressors and is defined as a minimal discrepancy between demands and capabilities (McCubbin et al., 1996). Family function is efforts to achieve a new level of balance and fit after a family crisis. Family health is related to the accomplishment of essential functions and tasks.

Measurement of the Resiliency Model of Family Stress, Adjustment, and Adaptation

Researchers usually used Family Inventory of Life Events and Changes, and Family Pressure Scale-Ethic to measure the family stressor and strains; and often used the Coping Health Inventory for Parents, F-COPES: Family Crisis Oriented Personal Evaluation Scales (McCubbin, Larson, & Olson, 1996), and Family Problem Solving Communication (McCubbin, McCubbin, & Thompson, 1986b) to measure the degree of the family coping strategies. Family Hardiness Index (McCubbin, McCubbin, & Thompson, 1986a), the Family Inventory of Resources for Management (McCubbin, Comeau, & Harkins, 1981), and Family Time and Routines Index (McCubbin, McCubbin, & Thompson, 1986) were often used to measure the characteristics of hardiness as a stress resistance and adaptation resource that refers to the internal strengths and durability of the family unit (McCubbin, Thompson et al., 1996). Family appraisal was measured using the Family Sense of Coherence (Antonovsky & Sourani, 1988). Family schema was measured using the Family (Ethnicity) Schema Index (McCubbin, Thompson, Elver, & Carpenter, 1992). Family cohesion was measured using the Family Adaptability and Cohesion Evaluation Scale. Family adaptation was measured using the Family Assessment Device (Epstein, Baldwin, & Bishop, 1983). Researcher listed nine instruments in Table 1, which would be used in examining the resilience of families with a disabled child and also compare the different instruments with theory, concepts, development of instruments and operationalization that was presented in Table 1.

After reviewing the psychometric data of the resiliency model of family stress, adjustment and adaptation, it can select the Family Index of Regenerativity and Adaptation-General (FIRA-G) as a measurement tool, which includes 74 items to evaluate the resilience of families of children with disabilities (McCubbin, 1987; McCubbin, Thompson et al., 1996). The reasons include that (a) the FIRA-G is an effort to develop a cluster of family measures designed and selected to assess the critical dimensions and components of the family stress model; (b) even though there are too many items in the FIRA-G, it can evaluate the seven dimensions of concepts that may tend to include both stages of the resilience model, adjustment and adaptation; (c) the other eight instruments can only measure one of the sub-concepts of the resilience model such as family stress, pile-up of demands, family resource, family appraisal or family function; but there are a lot of articles contributing to the knowledge of the individual concepts; (d) thirty seven of the major items of the FIRA-G are derived from the F-COPES which contains 30 items (McCubbin, Larson et al., 1996) and the FILE which contains 71 items (McCubbin, Patterson, & Wilson, 1983). The decrease in items is better able to match the ability of human concentration.

The FIRA-G can use the family system to view all the concepts; however, only a few articles have used the instrument to explore its validity and reliability because the instrument was so recently developed. McCubbin's group developed the resiliency model and established a lot of instruments, which expanded the knowledge of other concepts, but did not help to develop the knowledge of family resilience. The FIRA-G does not include family schema and family adaptation; so, in the future I would like to add the Family Assessment Device and the Family Schema-Ethic Index to explore the correlation between family resilience and family function to develop the knowledge of family resilience.

References

Antonovsky, A., & Sourani, T. (1988). Family sense of coherence and family adaptation. *Journal of Marriage and the Family, 50,* 79-92.

Atkin, K., & Ahmad, W. I. U. (2000). Family care-giving and chronic illness: How parents cope with a child a sickle cell disorder or thalassaemia. *Health and Social Care in the Community, 8,* 57-69.

Bennett, T., & DeLuca, D. A. (1996). Families of children with disabilities: Positive adaptation across the life cycle. *Social Work in Education, 18,* 31- 44.

Braverman, M. T. (2001). applying resilience theory to the prevention of adolescent substance abuse. *Focus, Spring*(1-12).

Brown, L. (1993). *The new shorter Oxford English Dictionary on historical principles* (Vol. 2). Oxford: Clarendon.

Cohen, O., Slonim, I., Finzi, R., & Leichtentritt, R. D. (2002). Family resilience: Israeli mothers' perspectives. *American Journal of Family Therapy, 30,* 173-187.

Dyson, L. L. (1997). Fathers and mothers of school-age children with developmental disabilities: Parental stress, family functioning and social support. *American Journal on Mental Retardation, 102,* 267-279.

Epstein, N., Baldwin, L., & Bishop, D. (1983). The McMaster family assessment device. *Journal of Marital and Family Therapy, 9,* 17 1- 180.

Failla, S., & Jones, L. C. (1991). Families of children with developmental disabilities: An examination of family hardiness. *Research in Nursing & Health, 14,* 41-50.

Flexner, S. B., & Hauck, L. C. (1993). *Random house unabridged dictionary.* New York: Rndom house.

Gottlieb, A. (1998). Single mother of children with disabilities: the role of sense of coherence in managing multiple challenges. In H. I. McCubbin & E. A. Thompson & A. I. Thompson & J. E. Fromer (Eds.), *Stress, coping, and health in families: sense of coherence and resilience* (pp. 189-206). Thousand Oaks, CA: Sage.

Hawley, D., & De Haan, L. (1996). Towards a definition of family resilience: Integrating individual and family perspectives. *Family Process, 35,* 283-298.

Institue for Health and Disability. (1997). A new way to think about cultural sensitivity: Families share their understanding of disabilities. *Health Issues for Children & Youth and their family, 5*(1), 1-12.

Judge, S. L. (1998). Parental coping strategies and strengths in families of young childen with disabilities. *Family Relations, 47*, 262-267.

Kazak, A. E. (1992). The social context of coping with childhood chronic illness: Family systems and social support. In A. M. La Greca & et al (Eds.), *Stress and coping in child health*. New York: Guilford

Lustig, D. (1997). Families with an adult with mental retardation: Empirical family typologies. *Rehabilitation Counseling Bulletin, 41*, 138-157.

Margalit, M., & Yona, L. (1991). Community support in Israeli kibbutz and city families of children with disabilities: Family climate and parental coherence. *Journal of Special Education, 24*, 427-440.

Masten, A. S. (1994). Resilience in individual development: successful adaptation despite risk and adversity. In M. C. Wang & E. W. Gorden (Eds.), *Educational resilience in inner-city America* (pp. 3-25). Hillsdale, NJ: Erlbaum.

McCubbin, H. I. (1987). Family Index of Regenerativity and Adaptation-General (FIRA-G). In H. I. McCubbin & A. I. Thompson & M. A. McCubbin (1996), *Family assessment: Resiliency, coping, and adaptation- Inventories for research and practice* (pp. 823-842). Madison: University of Wisconsin System.

McCubbin, H. I., Comeau, J., & Harkins, J. (1981). Family Inventroy of Resources for Management (FIRM). In H. I. McCubbin & A. I. Thompson & M. A. McCubbin (1996), *Family assessment: Resiliency, coping, and adaptation- Inventories for research and practice* (pp. 307-324). Madison: University of Wisconsin System.

McCubbin, H. I., Larson, A., & Olson, D. (1996). Family crisis orient personal scales (F-COPES). In H. I. McCubbin & A. I. Thompson & M. A. McCubbin (1996), *Family assessment: Resiliency, coping and adaptation--intventories for research and practice* (pp. 455-508). Madison, WI: University of Wisconsin-Madison.

McCubbin, H. I., & McCubbin, M. A. (1988). Typologies of resilient families: Emerging roles of social class and ethnicity. *Family Relations, 37*, 247-259.

McCubbin, H. I., McCubbin, M. A., & Thompson, A. I. (1986). Family Time and Routines Index (FTRI). In H. I. McCubbin & A. I. Thompson & M. A. McCubbin (1996), *Family assessment: Resiliency, coping and adaptation-Inventories for research and practice* (pp. 325-340). Madison: University of Wisconsin System.

McCubbin, H. I., McCubbin, M. A., Thompson, A. I., & Thompson, E. I. (1998). Resiliency in ethic families: A conceptual model for predicting family adjustment and adaptation. In H. I. McCubbin & E. A. Thompson & A. I. Thompson & J. E. Fromer (1996), *Resiliency in Native American and immigrant families* (pp. 3-48). Thousand Oaks, CA: Sage.

McCubbin, H. I., & Patterson, J. M. (1983). Family transitions: Adaptation to stress. In H. I. McCubbin & C. R. Figley (Eds.), *Stress and the family: Vol. 1 Coping with normative transitions* (pp. 5-25). New York: Brunner/Mazel.

McCubbin, H. I., Patterson, J. M., & Wilson, L. (1983). Family Inventory of Life Events and Changes (FILE). In H. I. McCubbin & A. I. Thompson & M. A. McCubbin (1996), *Family assessment: Resiliency, coping and adaptation-Inventories for research and practice* (pp. 103-178). Madison: University of Wisconsin System.

McCubbin, H. I., Thompson, A. I., Elver, K., & Carpenter, K. (1992). Family Schema-Ethnic (FSCH-E). In H. I. McCubbin & A. I. Thompson & M. A. McCubbin. (1996), *Family assessment: Resiliency, coping and adaptation-Inventories for research and practice* (pp. 713-722). Madison: University of Wisconsin.

McCubbin, H. I., Thompson, A. I., & McCubbin, M. A. (1996). *Family assessment: Resiliency, coping and adaptation: Inventories for research and practice*. Madison, WI: University of Wisconsin Publisher.

McCubbin, H. I., Thompson, A. I., Thompson, E. A., Elver, K. M., & McCubbin, M. A. (1998). Ethnicity, schema, and coherence: Appraisal processes for families in crisis. In J. E. Fromer (Ed.), *Stress, coping, and health in families: Sense of coherence and resiliency* (pp. 41-67). Madison, WI: University of Wisconsin Press.

McCubbin, M. A., McCubbin, H. I., & Thompson, A. I. (1986a). Family Hardiness Index (FHI). In H. I. McCubbin & A. I. Thompson & M. A. McCubbin (1996), *Family assessment: Resiliency, coping and adaptation-Inventories for research and practice* (pp. 239-306). Madison: University of Wisconsin System.

McCubbin, M. A., McCubbin, H. I., & Thompson, A. I. (1986b). Family Problem Solving and Coping (FPSC). In H. I. McCubbin & A. I. Thompson & M. A. McCubbin (1996), *Family assessment: Resiliency, coping and adaptation-Inventories for research and practice* (pp. 639-686). Madison: University of Wisconsin System.

Olsen, S. F., Marshall, E. S., Mandleco, B. L., Allred, K. W., Dyches, T. T., & Sansom, N. (1999). Support, communication, and hardiness in families with children with disabilities. *Journal of Family Nursing, 8*, 275-291.

Patterson, J. M., & McCubbin, H. I. (1983). Chronic illness: Family stress and coping. In H. I. McCubbin (Ed.), *Stress and the family: Volume II: Coping with Catastrophe* (pp. 21-36). New York: Brunner/Mazel.

Robinson, M., & Davidson, G. (1996). *Chambers 21st Century Dictionary*. England: Chamber.

Silliman, B., & Pike, L. B. (2002). *Family resiliency factors commonly identified in research. In 1994 Resiliency research review: Conceptual & research foundations..* Retrieved February 15, 2002, from the World Wide Web: http://www.cyfernet.org/research/resilreview.htm

Walsh, F. (1998). *Strengthening family resilience*. New York: Guilford Press.

Walsh, F. (2002). A family resilience framework: innovative practice application. *Family Relations, 51*, 130-137.

Table 1 Major Components (Dimension) and Operationalization of the Family Resiliency Model

Authors and Resources	Dimensions / Concepts	Operationalization	Instruments	Instrument and Applied
McCubbin, H. I. Comeau, J. Harkins, J. (1981, 1996)	Family stressor / Pile up Family strengths I: Esteem and communication Family strengths II: Mastery and health Extended family social support Financial well-being Source of financial support Social desirability	Personal resources: financial, education, health, & psychological attributes Family system internal resources: family adaptability and family integration or cohesion, managerial ability, problem solving ability Social support: emotional support, network support, esteem support	Family Inventory of Resources for management (FIRM): 68 items, 0-3 scale	Children recently diagnosed with insulin-dependent diabetes mellitus (N=53), Cardiac surgery patient/spouse pairs 6 months after surgery (N=67). Families randomly selected from family practice clinics in Minnesota & University of Minnesota faculty & staff (N=124), Families coping with major vascular surgery & recovery (N=42), Single-parent families of children with cerebral palsy, matched to two-parent families based on severity of impairment (N=166), Families of previously healthy infants who had an emergency apnea episode & were subsequently placed on a home apnea monitor (N=30), Families raising preschoolers with developmental disabilities (N=16)
McCubbin, H. I. Patterson, J. Wilson, L. (1983)	Family stress / Pile-up	Stress arises from an accumulation of life events and plays a role in the etiology of various somatic and psychiatric disorders	Family Inventor of Life Event and Changes (FILE): 71 items Intrafamily strains Marital strains Pregnancy and childbearing strains Finance and business strains Work-family transitions and strains Illness and family care strains Losses	Families relocated to a new city in Texas within 2 years prior to the study (N=53), Parent dyads who had a son with learning disability & parent dyads who had a son with no academic difficulties (N=56), Women whose husbands were hospitalized for coronary by pass surgery & 6 weeks after discharge (N=86)

Authors and Resources	Dimensions / Concepts	Operationalization	Instruments	Instrument and Applied
			Transitions in and out Legal Family Pressure Scale-Ethic:	Parents of abused children (N=137) Families of children with heterogeneous brain tumors (N=63)
McCubbin, M. A. McCubbin, H. I. Thompson, A. I. (1986, 1996)	Family hardiness / Family Resource, regenerative type	Hardiness was shown to function as a resistance resource to buffer the effects of stressful life events and that had its greatest health preserving effect when stressful life events increased Developed to measure the characteristics of hardiness as a stress resistance and adaptation resource in families which would function as a buffer or mediating factor in mitigating the effects of stressors and demands, and a facilitation of family adjustment and adaptation over time	Family Hardiness Index (FHI) 20 items Co-oriented commitment Confidence Challenge, & Control Family Inventory of Resources for Management	Families of children with asthma (N=27); Individuals attending a meeting at farm union in rural midwest community (N=206); Caregivers of children with cognitive and physical disabilities (N=63), Families of varying race: Caucasian (78), Asian (49), Hawaiian (37), & mixed race; Native Hawaiian families (155); investment executives of a regional investment firm with branch offices in sixteen states, and their spouse (N=311); Female & male employees who are part of a longitudinal study of work, families & health(N=156) Families with a large nationally recognized insurance company (N=304)

Authors and Resources	Dimensions / Concepts	Operationalization	Instruments	Instrument and Applied
McCubbin, H. I. McCubbin, M. A. Thompson, A. I. (1986, 1996)	Family time & routines / Family resources Family Bonding Family Coherence Family Celebration Quality of Family Life	Parent-child togetherness, couple together, Child routines, Meal's together subscale, Family time together, Family chores routines, Relatives connection routines	Family Time and Routines Index (FTRI)	Caucasian students (N=408) Adolescents currently living in a remarried household (N=95) Families associated with a large nationally recognized insurance company (N=304) High school students from 2 public high schools in a south western state (N=253)
McCubbin, M. A. McCubbin, H. I. Thompson, A. (1988, 1996)	Family problem solving and coping Incendiary communication Affirming communication	Generalized ways of responding to family hardship and difficulties by creating a family environment or context of communication in which and through which family hardships and issues are addressed and resolved	Family Resource Scale Family problem solving and coping (FPSC): 10 items with a four Likert scale	Employees of a national insurance company (N=1399) Mothers of children with cardiac illness (N=107), Diabetes (N=72) time1 Fathers of children with cardiac illness (N=92), diabetes (N=62) time1 Families of Native Hawaiian Ancestry (N=184) Single-parent families of Native Hawaiian Ancestry (N=109) Two parent families of Native Hawaiian Ancestry (N=80) Rural bank employees (N=743) Spouse of rural bank employees (N=413) Investment executives (N=297) Spouse of investment executives (N=233)

Authors and Resources	Dimensions / Concepts	Operationalization	Instruments	Instrument and Applied
McCubbin, H. I. Olson, D. Larson, A. (1981)	Family coherence / Family resource, Regenerative type	Family Crisis Oriented Personal Evaluation is to identify problem solving and behavioral strategies utilized by families in difficult or problematic situations. The items focus on the two levels of interaction outlined in the resiliency model. Individual to family system and family to social environment	Family Crisis Oriented Personal Evaluation Scales (F-COPES): 30 items Acquiring Social Support Reframing Seeking Spiritual Support Mobilizing Family to Acquire and Accept Help Passive Appraisal Original: 71 items Family resource: Confidence in family problem solving, Reframing family problem, Family passivity; Social and community resource: church/ religious resource, extended families, friends, neighbors, community resources	Parent dyads who had a son with a learning disability & parent dyads who had a son with no academic difficulties (N=56) Families of 30-month old children with mental delay & no delay (N=52) Parents or guardians of kindergarten children at 10 public schools in a rural setting (N=116) Couple with one member having spinal cord injury, both English speaking & able to demonstrate 6th grade reading proficiency (N=17) Primary caregivers of Alzheimer's disease patients followed at the older adult and memory Disorders clinic at strong memory hospital or attending Alzheimer's Association support groups (N=91) Families with mentally retarded persons living at home (N=62)
McCubbin, H. I. Larson, A. Olson, D. (1982)	Family coherence / Family resource, Regenerative type	Families call upon their appraisal skills to manage stressful life events, strains, and changes	Family Coherence Index: 4 items Acceptance of stressful events, accepting difficulties, a positive appraisal of a problem, & having faith in God	
McCubbin, H. I. Patterson, J. M. (1982)	Family coherence / Family resource, Regenerative type		Family Index of Coherence (Family Index of Regenerativity and Adaptation-Military: 17 items	

Authors and Resources	Dimensions / Concepts	Operationalization	Instruments	Instrument and Applied
McCubbin, H. I. Thompson, A. Elver, K. Carpenter, K. (1992)	Family schema/ Family identity, values, beliefs, rules, and boundaries	Family has cultivated a sense of cultural and ethnic values, which is an important part of the family's identity	Family Schema-Ethnic Index (FSCH-E): 39 items, 4-point Likert scale Confidence Meaningfulness Manageability Comprehensibility	Native Hawaiian (N=141)
Epstein, N. B. Baldwin, L. B. Bishop, D. S. (1982)	Family adaptation / Problem solving Communication Roles Affective Responsiveness Affective Involvement Behavioral control General Functioning	FAD assess 6 dimensions of family functioning	Family Assessment Device (FAD): 53 items, 4-point Likert scale Problem solving Communication Roles Affective Responsiveness Affective Involvement Behavioral control General Functioning	N=294 came from a group of 112 families with a child in a psychiatric day hospital, with a member with a stroke rehabilitation unit, students in advanced psychological courses, and a member was an inpatient in an adult psychiatric hospital. Retirement adjustment of 178 couples in their sixties. 218 non-clinical families and 98 clinical families.
McCubbin, H. I. (1987, 1996)	Family Indices of regenerativity and adaptation Pile-up Family support Community support Family resources Regenerative type Adaptation	Family processes interact with individual family members' psychological and physiological processes in discernible and predictable ways. A cluster of family measures designed and selected to assess the critical dimensions and components of the family stress model	Family stressors: FILE (10 items) Family strains: FILE (10 items) Relative and friend support: FCOPES (8 items) Social support: SSI (17 items) Family coherence: FCOPES (4 items) Family hardiness: FHI (20 items) Family distress: FILE (5 items)	Family stressors, Family strains, Family coherence, & Family distress (1000 families) Social support (1036 military families) Family hardiness (304 families)

Psychometric properties of the Family Resilience's Instrument

Instrument Development of FIRA-G

For research on family transition, crises, and adaptation, McCubbin (1987) used the Resiliency Model of Family Stress, Adjustment, and Adaptation to guide the selection of indices or family system measures. The Family Index of Regenerativity and Adaptation-General (FIRA-G) Inventory was developed. The resilience Model family dimension includes family stressors, family strains, relative and friend support, social support, family coherence, family hardiness, and family distress. Individual concepts such as pile-up, family support, community support, family resources, regenerative type, and adaptation are outcomes of family dimensions.

McCubbin (1987) selected 25 items from primary instrument of "Family Inventory of Life Events and Changes (FILE)" which has 71 items and is formed into three dimensions: family stressors (10 items), family strains (10 items), and family distress (5 items). In addition, he also selected 12 items from original instrument of "Family Crisis Oriented Personal Evaluation Scales (F-COPES) which has 30 items and is divided into two dimensions, relative and friend support (8 items) and family coherence (4 items). McCubbing incorporated the whole primary instrument of "Family Hardiness Index," which has 20 items into the FIRA-G dimension of family hardiness. At last he modified the original instrument of Social Support Index to form dimension of social support in FIRA-G.

Reliability and validity of the FIRA-G

The psychometric properties of the Family Stressors Index include a validity coefficient (correlation with the original FILE) of .6. The psychometric properties of the Family Strain Index include a reliability index (internal reliability) .69 and a validity coefficient (correlation with original FILE) of .87. The psychometric properties of the Social Support Index include a reliability (internal reliability) index of .82 and a validity coefficient (correlation with the criterion of family well-being) of .40. The psychometric properties of the Relative and Friend support Index include a reliability (internal reliability index of .82 and validity coefficient (correlation with the original F-COPES) of .99. The psychometric properties of the Family Coherence Index include a reliability (internal reliability) index of .71 and a validity coefficient (correlation with the original F-COPES) of .80. Reviewing these seven subscales of reliability and validity (correlation with the original scales), the researcher chose to analyze and critique the F-COPES scale because its reliability and validity were appropriate. They have higher reliability except the factors stress and strains. In addition, a few articles reported by using of the FIRA-G.

Development of F-COPES

The original scale of F-COPES was designed to integrate family resources and the meaning of perception factors identified in family stress theory into coping strategies. McCubbin, Olson, & Larsen (1981) reviewed the literature relating to coping theory and research, as well as other instruments, such as Family Coping Inventory (FCI) (McCubbin, Boss, Wilson, & Dahl, 1981) and the Coping Health Inventory of Parents (CHIP)(McCubbin, McCubbin, Nevin, & Cauble, 1979); The steps in the construction of the instrument that had 49 items and developed using a convenience sample of 119 family members representing all stages of the life cycle.

Reliability and Validity of F-COPE

After the analysis, the number of the items was reduced to 30, and used factor analysis procedures to determine two dimensions, internal family coping patterns that composed three categories: confidence in problem solving (Cronbache α: .7), reframing family solving (Cronbache α: .64), and family passivity (Cronbache α: .66); and external family coping patterns that consisted five scales, church/ religious resources (Cronbache α: .87), extended family (Cronbache α: .86), friends (Cronbache α: .74), neighbors (Cronbache α: .79), community resources (Cronbache α: .7). The overall reliability for the entire instrument was (Cronbache α: .7).

Critical Comparison of the Findings of F-COPES

Factor analysis supported the five subscales structure. A sample (N=119) included undergraduate and graduate students. They selected 30 items that each item's factor loading was greater than .38 and eight factors had eigenvalues greater than one. So, the construct validity was good. The alpha reliability for the entire scale was .77 that a higher internal consistency. An additional sample (2582) was obtained and randomly split into two halves, sample 1 (1338) and sample 2 (1244). Factor analysis using varimax rotation identified five factors: acquiring social support, reframing, seeking spiritual support, mobilizing family to acquire and accept help, and passive appraisal. Alpha reliability of each factor and test-retest for final scale and the total scale are listed in table 1. Test-retest reliability was satisfactory except the subscale of reframing and passive appraisal. The time lapse of test-retest reliability between the first and second administration was four weeks that was appropriate.

These five structures have been used in all subsequent research. Among the five factors, the factors acquiring social support and reframing, had higher reliability. So, McCubbin (1987) selected 7 items from acquiring social support (9 items) renamed the category "relative and friend support (8 items)", and selected 3 items from reframing (8 items) renamed the category "family coping coherence". The factor passive appraisal had lower reliability and test-retest score. The factor reframing also had lower test-retest score more than another four factors.

McCubbin, Thompson, MaCubbin, Elver, Futrel, & Masshardt (1996) reviewed research involving the use of F-COPES, among the 94 published reports, there were only sixteen articles reported the reliability (.61-.96). Reliability in the forty doctoral dissertations and eighteen master theses are non-available. The scale that used different samples included (a) parents with learning disabilities, mental delay, kindergarten age children, cognitive or physical disabilities, serious illness; (b) couples with one member having spinal cord injury, breast cancer, and severe premenstrual symptom; (c) primary caregivers of Alzheimer's disease, cardiac arrest survivor, vascular surgery, head injury, cardiac transplantation, and chronic disease.

Samuelson, Foltz, and Foxall (1992) used a convenience sample of 17 families (34 parents) of preschool and school-age children with myelomeningocele: the family coping was measured using F-COPES (30 items, 5-point scale ranging from strongly disagree to strongly agree). Items were divided into eight subscales: confidence in problem-solving, reframing family problem, family passivity, spititual resources, extended family, friends, neighbors, and community resources. Reported alpha for the total scale is .77 with alpha ranging from.64 to .87 for the subscales. The Cronbache alpha of stressor and coping strategies for mother was .76 and for father was .85. The alpha showed higher internal consistency. The mothers had higher mean score on the total coping score on the total coping scale than fathers. The researchers never verified the validity; they just used the content validity that was reported by McCubbin et al (1987).

Worden and Silverman (1993) used a community-based sample of seventy bereaved families with school age children who were assessed four months after the death and at the first anniversary by F-COPES. The scale of F-COPES including 29 items and six different scales was different from McCubbin's et al F-COPES. The researchers did not describe the modification. The alpha reliabilities were ranging from .64 to .87 and acceptable, test-retest reliabilities from .49 to .85. And the result present eight scales, so I think six scales may be a mistake.

Dougherty (1995) used fifteen sudden cardiac arrest survivors to assess their family coping by using of F-COPES. Internal consistency reliabilities were ranging from .71 to .87 for the subscale and for the total scale were .87 for survivors and .81 for spouses. The researcher never described the content or construct validity.

In general, construct validation on extreme groups was investigated. Internal consistency was appropriate. Test-retest reliability and construct validity was good. Referrer F-COPES scores predicted family coping in facing stressors or referral suitability. Sensitivity to change requires further investigation. The F-COPES can be recommended for use by all agencies but need to modify for different situations because the verified construct content had five or eight factors.

References

McCubbin, H. I. (1987). Family Index of Regenerativity and Adaptation-General (FIRA-G). In H. I. McCubbin & A. I. Thompson & M. A. McCubbin (Eds.), *Family assessment: Resiliency, coping, and adaptation- Inventories for research and practice* (pp. 823-842). Madison: University of Wisconsin System.

McCubbin, H. I., Boss, P., Wilson, L., & Dahl, B. (1981). Family Coping Inventory. In H. I. McCubbin & A. I. Thompson (Eds.), *Family assessment for research and practice* (pp. 219-232). Madison: University of Wisconsin-Madison.

McCubbin, H. I., Larsen, A. S., & Olson, D. H. (1982a). Family Coping Coherence Index. In H. I. McCubbin & A. I. Thompson & M. A. McCubbin (Eds.), *Family assessment: Resiliency, coping and adaptation-Inventories for research and practice* (Vol. 703-712). Madison: University of Wisconsin System.

McCubbin, H. I., Larsen, A. S., & Olson, D. H. (1982b). Relative and Friend Support. In H. I. McCubbin & A. I. Thompson & M. A. McCubbin (Eds.), *Family assessment: Resiliency, coping and adaptation-Inventories for research and practice* (pp. 835). Madison: University of Wisconsin System.

McCubbin, H. I., McCubbin, M. A., Nevin, R., & Cauble, A. E. (1979). Family assessment for research and practice. In H. I. McCubbin & A. I. Thompson (Eds.), *1987* (pp. 181-199). Madison: Univesity of Wisconcin-Madison.

McCubbin, H. I., Olson, D. H., & Larson, A. S. (1981). Family Crisis Oriented Personal Evaluattion Scale. In H. I. McCubbin & A. I. Thompson & M. A. McCubbin (Eds.), *Family assessment: Resiliency, coping, and adaptation-Inventories for research and practice* (pp. 455-508). Madison: University of Wisconsin System.

McCubbin, H. I., & Patterson, J. M. (1982). Family Strains. In H. I. McCubbin & A. I. Thompson & M. A. McCubbin (Eds.), *Family assessment: Resiliency, coping and adaptation-Inventories for research and practice* (pp. 834). Madison: University of Wisconsin System.

McCubbin, H. I., Patterson, J. M., & Glynn, T. (1982). Social Support Index. In H. I. McCubbin & A. I. Thompson & M. A. McCubbin (Eds.), *Family assessment: Resiliency, coping and adaptation-Inventories for research and practice* (pp. 357-390). Madison: University of Wisconsin System.

McCubbin, H. I., Patterson, J. M., & Wilson, L. (1983). Family Inventory of Life Events and Changes (FILE). In H. I. McCubbin & A. I. Thompson & M. A. McCubbin (Eds.),

Family assessment: Resiliency, coping and adaptation-Inventories for research and practice (pp. 103-178). Madison: University of Wisconsin System.

McCubbin, M. A., McCubbin, H. I., & Thompson, A. I. (1986). Family Hardiness Index (FHI). In H. I. McCubbin & A. I. Thompson & M. A. McCubbin (Eds.), *Family assessment: Resiliency, coping and adaptation-Inventories for research and practice* (pp. 239-306). Madison: University of Wisconsin System.

Samuelson, J. J., Foltz, J., & Foxall, M. J. (1992). Stress and coping in families of children with myelomeningocele. *Archieves of psychiatric Nursing, 4*, 287-295.

Warden, J. W., & Silverman, P. S. (1993). Grief and depression in newly widowed parents with school-age children. *Omega, 27*, 251-261.

Psychometric Properties of the Family Assessment Device

The Family Assessment Device (FAD) is designed to permit clinicians and researchers to screen for health and pathology of family functioning on a variety of clinically relevant dimensions. The development of FAD, a 53-item, self-report scale was designed to assess seven dimensions, which are based on the McMaster Model of Family Function (Epstein, Baldwin, & Bishop, 1982). The McMaster Model is based on systems, role, and communication theories, and evolved from work with non-clinical families (Sawin & Harrigan, 1995). In order to represent the complexities of a family, the model identified six dimensions: Problem Solving, Communication, Roles, Affective Responsiveness, Affective Involvement, and Behavior Control. Six of the scales on the FAD reflected the dimensions of family functioning outlined in the McMaster Model of Family Functioning (Epstein, Bishop, & Levin, 1978). Additionally, Epstein, Baldwin, and Bishop (1983) selected the items most highly intercorrelated, which resulted in the creation of a General Functioning dimension, which assessed overall health-pathology of family.

The present study reports of the FAD consisted of 60 items (with seven items added to three of the scales to increase reliability of the original 53-item version) (Bernstein, Garbin, & McClellan, 1983). The scales and dimensions of the FAD included: six items for Problem Solving, nine items for Communication, 11 items for Roles, six items for Affective Responsiveness, seven items for Affective Involvement, nine items for Behavior Control, and 12 items for General Functioning. The General Functioning can be used independently from the other scales as an over-all measures (Epstein et al., 1982). This paper will explore the psychometric properties of the FAD including reliability and validity, ethical problems, cultural sensitivity, critic, and related studies using the FAD.

Psychometric Properties of FAD

Reliability

Internal Consistency. A sample of 503 individuals made of 294 clinical members from 112 families and 209 non-clinical introductory psychology students. The psychometric properties of the FAD included a reliability index (internal reliability) .72 to .92. The seven scales were moderately correlated (.37-.67), but the partial correlations approached zero when the General Functioning scale was held constant (Epstein, et al., 1983). Subsequent reports consistently supported internal stability of all scales but the Roles scale (Kabacoff, Miller, Bishop, Epstein, & Keitner, 1990; Miller, Epstein, Bishop, & Keitner, 1985). The lower reliabilities have been obtained for non-clinical samples, thus the Roles scale should be used cautiously, especially with non-clinical samples.

Kabacoff, et al. (1990) recruited sample from psychiatric hospital, medical outpatient clinic, and non-clinical to investigate their family function used the FAD, which included 627 non-clinical persons, 1138 psychiatric patients, and 298 medical patients. They get moderate to high reliability (Cronbach alpha: .7-.86) except Role dimension among the three groups. In addition, they compare reliability of FAD-item 53 that could not find the higher reliability among the three groups for dimension of Problem Solving, Communication, and Roles.

Test-Retest. The test-retest estimates of the FAD were over a one-week period (N=45 non-clinical individuals). The correlation coefficients were adequate: Problem Solving, .66; communication, .72; Roles, .75; Affective Responsiveness, .76; Affective Involvement, .67; Behavior Control, .73; and General Functioning, .71 (Browne, Arpin, Coey, Fitch, & Gafni, 1990; Miller et al., 1985). Browne, Arpin, Coey, Fitch, and Gafni (1990) reported similar test-retest data. .

Validity

Construct Validity. Kabacoff et al. (1990) used confirmatory factor analyses that provided support for the structure of the FAD. Coefficient of factor invariance indicated that the FAD has higher similar structure in non-clinical, psychiatric, and medical samples. The fact that the FAD was not developed through factor analytic methods (Epstein, Baldwin, & Bishop, 1983), over 90 % of FAD items loaded on factors hypothesized by McMaster Model. The confirmatory factors accounted for test variance that the amount of variance accounted for (37%) by a six-factors principle component model. It seems rather low. Kabacoff, et al. (1990) described that the FAD appeared to correspond well to the hypothesized theoretical structure from the McMaster Model after they compared the amount of variance accounted for in principle components analysis of other self-report family assessment measures such as the Family Concept Test (VanderVeen & Olson, 1981) and the Family Environment Scale (Fowler, 1981). I can't agree with that view of comparing different accounted variance among the different instruments. However, they were also low for the amount of accounted variance among the instruments.

Concurrent Validity. Preliminary evidence for the validity of the FAD consisted of: (a) discrimination between psychiatric and non-clinical families, and (b) prediction of morale in a sample of retired couples (Epstein, et al., 1983). Epstein et al. (1983) used a sample of 45 non-clinical individuals to assess the concurrent validity of the FAD by administering the

FAD, Family Adaptability and Coherence Evaluation Scales II, and Family Unit Inventory (FUI) to these subjects. The obtained relationships between the FAD and the FUI provided adequate evidence of concurrent validity of the FAD. Lower correlations were reported between the Family Integration and the Roles and Behavior Control Scales of the FAD. For the FUI Coping scale, the predicted relationship between the Coping scales and the FAD Communication scale was evidenced.

Miller, Kabacoff, Epstein, Bishop, Keitner, Baldwin, and van der Spuy (1994) explored FAD score of 93 depressed inpatients and their families, and found FAD and the McMaster Clinical Rating Scale (MCRS) correlated significantly (.4-.6) all scales except Behavior Control. Fristad (1989) found significant correlation among all dimensions of FAD and MCRS except Affective Responsiveness that were administered by 41 families of a mixed group of psychiatric patients and outpatients. The significant correlations (.40-.60) between most of the scales of the MCRS and the FAD indicate a moderate level of overlap between these two methods for measuring the dimensions of the McMaster Model. The obtained results may be due to inadequacies in the MCRS and FAD. They do not have sufficient data to determine which alternatives best explain the current data because of the consistent relationship found with the Behavior Control dimension and Affective Responsiveness (Miller et al., 1994). The FAD has been found to have low correlations with Social Desirability (r = .06-.19), moderate correlations with global measures of marital functioning such as the Dyadic Adjustment scale and the Locke-Wallace Marital Satisfaction scale (r = .47, .59), and theoretical consistent correlations with other measures of family functioning (Miller et al., 1985). The Social Desirability scale does not appear a strong influence on FAD scores.

Discriminant Validity. Keitner, Miller, Ryan, Epstein, and Bishop (1989) found that the mean of FAD difference between patients with either only depression or depression and at least one other psychiatric diagnosis. Keitner, Ryan, Fodor, and Miller (1990) presented the mean of FAD difference between Hungarians (N=58 non-clinical families) and North Americans (N=98 non-clinical families). Individuals' FAD scores for 218 non-clinical families and 98 clinical families were used in a discriminant analysis to predict whether the family came from clinical or non-clinical groups. The result presented that the non-clinical mean was lower than the mean for the clinically presenting group (Epstein, et al., 1983).

The FAD scales for adaptability correlate too highly with its Cohesion scale and present the most serious problems with discriminant validity. The Cohesion scale on the FAD

(Affective Involvement (AFF IN)) yields a higher correlation with the adaptability dimension on the SFIS-R (Mother-Child Cohesion/ Estrangement (MCC/E), Father-Child Cohesion/ Estrangement (FCC/E), and Spouse Conflict Resolved/Unresolved (SPCON R/U)); only in the case of the AFF IN scales on the FAD and the Enmeshment / Disengagement (EN/D) scales on the SFIS-R is the correlation between Cohesion scales higher than between Cohesion and Adaptability Scales. Two of the Adaptability scales on the FAD (Behavior Control and Roles) correlated higher with some of the cohesion scales on the SFIS-R than with the Adaptability scales on the SFIS-R; only in the case of the Problem Solving scale on the FAD and the Flexibility/Rigidity scale on the SFIS-R is the correlation between the Adaptability and Cohesion scales. Discriminant validity also fails to hold up between the FAD and the FES as well as between the FES, the FAD and the Family Adaptability and Cohesion Evaluation (FACES III). Discriminant validity is weakened by flaws particularly with the FAD (Perosa & Perosa, 1990).

Sawyer, Sarris, Baghurst, Cross, and Kalucy (1988) compared responses on the FAD obtained from healthy and clinical 94 families that consisted of mothers, fathers, and adolescents. Members of the clinic families consistently rated their families as less healthy than did families in the community. Adolescents in both groups of families rated their families as significantly less healthy than their parents. The results of the study provide support for the discriminative validity of the FAD between families containing an adolescent member referred to a mental health service and families containing an adolescent, living in community.

Predictor Validity. Epstein et al (1983) used regression analysis to assess concurrent validity from a random sample of 178 couples in their sixties. The FAD predicted 28% of the variance on the Locke Wallace Marital Satisfaction Scale, and predicted 22% of variance in the Moral Scores for husbands and 17% of variance for wives. The FAD was the more powerful predictor. Keitner, Ryan, Miller, and Norman (1992) indicated that family functioning assessed by the FAD was one of the five best predictors of recovery from a depressive episode. FAD was the strongest predictor of the total number of days re-hospitalized after stroke rehabilitation, accounting for 37% of the variance (Evans, Bishop, & Haselkorn, 1991).

Convergent Validity. The convergent validity of the adaptability scales is less promising, chiefly for the FAD Behavior Control and Role scales. The pairs of correlations between the FAD Behavior Control, Problem Solving, and Roles Scales with each of the adaptability scales on the other measures are much lower, ranging from .07 between Roles and the FACES III Adaptability scales to .61 between the Problem Solving scales and the Structural Family Interaction Scale-Revised (SFIS-R) Flexibility/ Rigidity scale. The intercorrelations among pairs of FAD Adaptability scales is higher, ranging from .47 between the Behavior Control and Problem Solving scales to .63 for Problem Solving and Roles (Perosa & Perosa, 1990).

Summary of Studies using the FAD

The FAD has been used with families responding to the demands of a variety of psychiatric problems that included alcohol dependence, depression, affective disorders, schizophrenia, adjustment, mental retardation, and bipolar disorders It has been used in clinical studies of families responding to adolescent suicide and other mental health issues. As well as it has been used with families responding to the demands of a wide range of medical problems that included systemic lupus, traumatic brain injury, stroke, rheumatoid arthritis, spinal cord injury, Parkinson's disease, and other disabilities (Sawin & Harrigan, 1995). It has been translated into fourteen languages, with evidence of its utility in different cultures (Keitner, Ryan, Miller et al., 1990; Keitner, Ryan, Miller, Kohn, & Epstein, 1991; Morris, 1990; Wenniger, Hageman, & Arrindell, 1993) and has been used in over forty research studies. These studies supported the discriminative validity of the FAD and its utility as a research instrument.

Some researchers reported that the McMaster model family assessment correlated well with observational measures of family functioning and was related to current maternal illness (Dickstein et al., 1998; Hayden et al., 1998; Max et al., 1998; Max et al., 1997). The FAD has also been used in investigations of children with psychiatric inpatients (McKay, Murphy, Rivinus, & Maisto, 1991), ADHD (Cunningham, Benness, & Siegel, 1988), and outpatients at a child psychiatric clinic (Goodyear, Nicol, Eavis, & Pollinger, 1982). The FAD can be used as a screening assessment to identify families, which are having problems, particular areas of difficulty within the family, and to assess change in families following treatment.

Ethical Consideration

Based on respecting for persons, beneficence, and justice that includes all persons should have autonomy and self-determination. That autonomy is reduced because of age, illness, or incapacity is enabling to protection. It is particular important for supporting subjects' rights to informed consent. The principle is not only to the duty not to harm others, but also to the duty to maximize potential benefits and minimize possible risks associated with the research or measurement procedure. It is important for providing subjects' right to protection from harm and for analyzing the ratio of potential risks to benefits. The principle of justice refers to the obligation to treat individuals equally and fairly.

According these basic ethical dimensions of measurement activities include informed consent, refusal to participate or withdrawal without recrimination, privacy, confidentiality and anonymity and protection from harm. Essential elements of informed consent are competence to consent, disclosure of information, subjects' understanding of the information, voluntaries of the consent, and authorization of consent. Researcher needs to provide information including a description of the research and its purpose, procedures, time and energy required, confidentiality provisions, any discomforts, risks and benefits. Subjects is given explicit instruction that participation is voluntary, withdrawal from or discontinuation of participation is possible without prejudice, and benefits will not be affected by participation (Waltz, Strickland, & Lens, 1991) measurement in nursing research.

A measure of instrument or activity may inadvertently expose the subject to stress resulting from loss of self-esteem, generation of self-doubt, embarrassment, guilt, disturbing self-insights, fright, or concern about things of which the subject was previously unaware. Subjects such as mothers of young children may be unable to participate in time-consuming measurement procedures such as in-depth interviews. Subjects who are ill or under stress are particularly vulnerable to risk of fatigue and should not be expected to engage in lengthy sessions or physically demanding activities.

Culturally Sensitive Family Assessment

Morris (1990) reported that the FAD appeared to make appropriate assessments of Hawaiian-American study participants' families and inappropriate assessments of Japanese-American study participants' families. The results suggested that cultural norms regarding family functioning might vary according to socioeconomic status. The FAD assessed Japanese-American families as having an extremely constricted range of emotions and inappropriate emotional responses. he norms of the FAD incorrectly assessed the emotional response of Japanese-American participants' families as unhealthy. Further, similar studies of ethnic subgroups are a more likely research strategy for building a knowledge base on the cultural sensitivity of instruments like the FAD. Using the FAD with an ethnically varied client population will make family practitioners more effective and relevant in modern, multi-cultural societies.

Critique Summary of The FAD

A particular strength of the FAD is the number of languages in which the instrument is available, making it possible to study and compare families from a variety of cultures. The need for psychometric data to be established with different cultural populations is recognized and currently underway. The FAD has been found to have high levels of internal consistency across a variety of different types of families (Epstein et al., 1983), and acceptable levels of test-retest reliability (Browne et al., 1990; Miller et al., 1985). But internal consistency was lower for the Roles scale (Kabacoff et al., 1990). The lowest reliabilities have been obtained for nonclinical samples, thus the Role scale should be used very cautiously (Kabacoff et al., 1990; Miller et al., 1985). Inter-rater reliability was not applicable.

Confirmatory factor analysis has supported the hypothesized underlying model of the FAD (Kabacoff et al., 1990). The construct validity was appropriate, but the amount of variance did not account for much. Ridenour et al., (1999, 2000) recommended that the FAD should be reorganized because they found two overseeing factors, Connection and Commitment, fit the FAD better than the McMaster's model. They indicated that best and most conservative use of the FAD is using the General Functioning subscale as a summary score (Ridenour, 1999). Miller et al. (2000) proposed that suggestion was premature and based on the inappropriate application of an internal consistency model of scale construction to the FAD. In the absence of this kind of data regarding alternative organizations of the FAD, Miller et al. (2000) believe that the original subscales remain the best choice. More research is necessary to determine if and how the FAD should be reorganized. There is much room for future research and increased knowledge concerning the FAD and its organization.

The predicted relationship between the scales of the FAD, FACES and the FUI provided adequate evidence of the concurrent validity for the FAD (Van der Veen et al., 1981). Regression analysis was used to test FAD with the Geriatric Morale Scale and the Locke Wallace Marital Satisfaction Scale (Epstein et al., 1983). The results indicated that the FAD was a more powerful predictor than was the Locke Wallace for morale. Family functioning also predicted the course of recovery for the stroke victims and was significantly related to major depression recovery prognosis (Keitner, Ryan, Miller, & Norman, 1992).

Sensitive information affects strong personal emotional responses from subjects, such as embarrassment, fear, stigma, guilt, anger, vulnerability, pain, stress, and anxiety; as well as sudden violent, death of a loved one, legal incarceration, and life-threatening illness, which are generally identified as sensitive topics. Other topics such as abortion, drug abuse, and controversial political activities may be viewed as more-or-less sensitive depending upon the specific attributes of subjects.

Shek (2001) examined the reliability and validity of the Chinese version of the General Function scale of Chinese FAD that has high test-retest reliability and internal consistency in different adolescent samples. These findings support the reliability of the GF scale. Shek (2001) suggested that the "GF scale of the Chinese FAD has acceptable psychometric properties and can be regard as instrument that can be used objectively by clinical practitioners to assess family perceptions in Chinese adolescents (p. 1512)." Because Shek found significantly correlated with other translated measures of family function that support concurrent validity and construct validity of the GF scale in different adolescent samples and the GF scores were able to differentiate participants from clinical and non-clinical families. The research finding needed a replication to assess the generalizability in different Chinese communities and expands to measure perceptions of the parents and late adolescents. As well as other methods of assessment such as observation and interview can be included to understand the group discriminate validity of the GF scale of the FAD, and examine the construct discriminant validity of the scale. Based on this reason I would like to select the General Function Scale as instrument in my future study.

References

Bernstein, L., Garbin, C., & McClellan, P. (1983). A confirmatory factoring of the California Psychological inventory. *Educational and Psychological Measurement, 43*, 687-691.

Browne, G. B., Arpin, K., Coey, P., Fitch, M., & Gafni, A. (1990). Prevalence and correlates of family dysfunction and poor adjustment to chronic illness in specially clinics. *Journal of Clinical Epidemiology, 43*, 373-383.

Cunningham, C., Benness, B., & Siegel, L. (1988). Family functioning, time allocation, and parental depression in the families of normal and ADDH children. *Journal of Clinical Child Psychology, 17*, 169-177.

Dickstein, S., Seifer, R., Hayden, I., Schiller, M., Sameroff, A. J., Keitner, G. I., Miller, I. V., Rasmussen, S., Matzko, M., & Magee, K. (1998). Levels of family assessment II: Impact of maternal psychopathology on family functioning. *Journal of Family Psychology, 12*, 23-34.

Epstein, N. B., Baldwin, L. B., & Bishop, D. S. (1982). McMaster Family Assessment Device, Version 3. In H. D. Grotevant & C. I. Carlson (Eds.), *Family assessment: A guide to methods and measures.* (pp. 340-343). New York: Guilford.

Epstein, N. B., Baldwin, L. M., & Bishop, D. S. (1983). The Mcmaster Family Assessment Device. *Journal of Marriage and Family Therapy, 9*, 171-180.

Epstein, N. B., Bishop, D. S., & Levin, S. (1978). The McMaster Model of Family Functioning. *Journal of Marriage and Family Counseling, 4*, 19-31.

Evans, R., Bishop, D. S., & Haselkorn, J. (1991). Factors predicting satisfactory home care after stroke. *Archieves of Physical Medicine and Rehabilitation, 72*, 1411-1413.

Fowler, R. (1981). Maximum likelihood factor structure of the family environment scale. *Journal of Clinical Psychology, 37*, 160-164.

Fristad, M. A. (1989). A comparison of the McMaster and Circumplex family assessment instrumenta. *Journal of Marital and Family Therapy, 15*, 259-269.

Goodyear, I., Nicol, R., Eavis, D., & Pollinger, G. (1982). Application and utility of a family assessment procedure in a child psychiaric clinic. *Journal of Family Therapy, 4*, 373-395.

Hayden, L., Schiller, M., Dickstein, S., Seifer, R., Sameroff, A. J., Miller, I. V., Keitner, G. I., & Rasmussen, S. (1998). Levels of family assessment 1: Family, marital and parent-child interaction. *Journal of Family Psychology, 12*, 7-22.

Kabacoff, R. I., Miller, I. W., Bishop, D. S., Epstein, N. B., & Keitner, G. I. (1990). A psychometric study of the McMaster family assessment device in psychiatric, medical, and nonclinical samples. *Journal of Family Psychology, 3*, 431-439.

Keitner, G. I., Miller, I. W., Ryan, C. E., Epstein, N. B., & Bishop, D. S. (1989). Compounded depression and family functioning during the acute episode and at 6-month follow-up. *Comprehensive Psychiatry, 30*, 512-521.

Keitner, G. I., Ryan, C. E., Fodor, J., & Miller, I. W. (1990). A cross-cultural sudy of family functioning. *Contemporary Family Therapy, 122*, 439-454.

Keitner, G. I., Ryan, C. E., Miller, I. V., Epstein, N. B., Bishop, D. S., & Norman, W. H. (1990). Family functioning, social adjustment and recurrence of suicidality. *Psychiatry, 53*, 17-30.

Keitner, G. I., Ryan, C. E., Miller, I. V., Kohn, R., & Epstein, N. B. (1991). 12-month outcome of patients with major depression and comorbid psychiatric or medical illness. *American Journal of Psychiatry, 148*, 345-350.

Keitner, G. I., Ryan, C. E., Miller, I. W., & Norman, W. H. (1992). Recovery and major depression factors associated with twelve-month outcome. *American Journal of Psychiatry, 143*, 93-99.

Max, J. E., Castillo, C. C., Robin, D. A., Lindgren, S. D., Smith, W. L., Sato, Y., Mattheis, P. J., & Stierwalt, J. A. (1998). Predictors of family functioning after traumatic brain injury in children and adolescents. *Journal of American Academy of Child & Adolescent Psychiatry, 37*, 83-90.

Max, J. E., Robinson, D. A., Lindren, S., Smith, D., Sato, M., Mattheis, P. J., Stierwalt, J. A., & Castillo, C. C. (1997). Traumatic brain injury in children and adolescents: Psychiatric disorders at two years. *Journal of American Academy of Child & Adolescent Psychiatry, 36*, 1278-1285.

McKay, J., Murphy, R., Rivinus, T., & Maisto, S. (1991). Family dysfunction and alcohol and drug use in adolescent psychiatric inpatients. *Journal of American Academy of Child & Adolescent Psychiatry, 30*, 967-972.

Miller, I. V., Epstein, N. B., Bishop, D. S., & Keitner, G. I. (1985). The McMaster Family Assessment Device: Reliability and validity. *Journal of Marital and Family Therapy, 11*, 345-356.

Miller, I. V., Kabacoff, R. I., Epstein, N. B., Bishop, D. S., Keitner, G. I., Baldwin, L. M., & van der Spuy, H. I. J. (1994). The development of a clinical rating scale for the McMaster model of family functioning. *Family Process, 33*, 53-69.

Miller, I. W., Bishop, D. S., Epstein, N. B., & Keitner, G. I. (1990). A psychometric study of the McMaster family assessment device in psychiatric, medical, and nonclinical samples. *Journal of Family Psychology, 3*, 431-439.

Miller, I. W., Ryan, C. E., Keitner, G. I., Bishop, D. S., & Epstein, N. B. (2000). Commentary "Factors analysis of the family assessment device" by Ridenour, Daley, & Reich. *Family Process, 39*, 141-144.

Morris, T. M. (1990). Culturally sensitive family assessment: an evaluation of the family assessment device with Hawaiian-American and Japanese-American families. *Family Process, 29*, 105-116.

Perosa, L. M., & Perosa, S. L. (1990). Convergent and discriminant validity for family self-report measures. *Educational and Psychological Measurement, 50*, 855-868.

Ridenour, T. A., Daley, J. G., & Reich, W. (1999). Factors analyses of the family assessment device. *Family Process, 38*, 497-510.

Sawin, K. J., & Harrigan, M. P. (1995). *Measures of family functioning for research and practice*. New York: Springer.

Sawyer, M. G., Sarris, A., Baghurst, P. A., Cross, D. G., & Kalucy, R. S. (1988). Family assessment device: reports from mothers, fathers, and adolescents in community and clinic families. *Journal of Marital and Family Therapy, 14*, 287-296.

Shek, D. T. L. (2001). The general function scale of the family assessment device: Does it work with chinese adolescents. *Journal of Clinical Psychology, 57*, 1503-1516.

VanderVeen, F., & Olson, R. (1981). Manual and handbook for the family concept assessment method. *Unpublished manuscript*.

Waltz, C. F., Strickland, O. L., & Lens, E. R. (1991). *Measurement in nursing research*. Philadelphia: F. A. Davis.

Wenniger, W., Hageman, W., & Arrindell, W. (1993). Cross-national validity of dimensions of family functioning: first experiences with the Dutch version of the McMaster family assessment device. *Personality and individual differences, 14*, 769-781.

Table 2 Major Components (Dimension) and Operationalization of the Family Resiliency Model

Instruments and Sources	Theory	Purpose/ Population/ Intention/ How did they come up with the concept	Dimensions / Concepts	Operationalization
Family Inventory of Resources for management (FIRM): 69 items 4-point scale McCubbin, H. I. Comeau, J. Harkins, J. (1981, 1996) In H. I. McCubbin, A.I. Thompson, M. A. McCubbin (Eds). Family Assessment: Resiliency, coping, and adaptation: Inventories for research and practice (p.). Madison, WI:University of Wisconsin	Resiliency Model of Family Stress, Adjustment, & Adaptation	Attempt to assess the family's repertoire of resources In order to describe or predict how a family adapts to stressful events, Call for information about which resources a family has, does not have, or has depleted. Firm was influenced by literature and theory in three major areas: **personal resources**—include financial, education, health, and psychological attributes; **family system internal resources**— family adaptability and family integration or cohesion, **social support**—emotional support, esteem support, and network support. Four subscribes derived from factors analytic procedures were used on the data from 322 families with a chronically ill child. Initial instrument included 98 self-reported items, four scales representing perceived family resources, the other two subscales are not considered major dimensions and not included in the factor analysis, but added to give the investigator additional information.	Family stressor / Pile up Family strengths I : Esteem and communication Family strengths II: Mastery and health Extended family social support Financial well-being Source of financial support Social desirability	69 items, evaluate on a 0-3 scale, four subscales: Family strengths 1—**Esteem and communication** (15 items), reflect the presence of a combination of personal, family system and social support resources in family esteem, communication, mutual assistance optimism, problem solving ability and encouragement of autonomy among family members; Family strengths II—**Mastery and health** (20 items), reflect personal, family system, and social support resources along sense of mastery over family events and outcomes family mutuality, and physical emotional health; **Extended family social support** (4 items), indicated the mutual help and support given to and received from relatives; education, health, & psychological attributes; **Financial well-being** (16 items), reflect the family's perceived financial efficacy; ability to meet financial commitments, adequacy of financial reserves, ability to help others, optimism about the family's financial future. **Sources of financial support** (7 items), reflect the sense of ability and esteem associated with income; **Social desirability** (7 items): are not considered part of the FIRM. Based on the Edmonds scale of marital conventionalization.

Instruments and Sources	Theory	Purpose/ Population/ Intention/ How did they come up with the concept	Dimensions / Concepts	Operationalization
Family Inventor of Life Event and Changes (FILE): 71 items McCubbin, H. I. Patterson, J. Wilson, L. (1980, 1983, 1996) McCubbin HI, Patterson J, Wilson L. Family Inventory of Life Events Scale (FILE). St. Paul: Univ. of Minnesota, Department of Family Social Services; 1982. McCubbin, H. I., Thompson, A. I., & McCubbin, M. A. (2001). *Family measures: Stress, coping, and resiliency – Inventories for research and practice.* Honolulu, Hawaii: Kamehameha Schools	Family stress theory	Developed as an index of family stress Assess the pile-up of life events Experienced by a family Applied the cumulative life changes in a systematic manner to the study of family behavior in response to stress Systematic method of inquiry was applied to the family in an effort to quantitatively document the impact of family life events and changes on the family system and individual members. Based on data from a sample of 322 families who have a chronically ill child (myelomeningocele or cerebral palsy)	Family stress / Pile-up Stress arises from an accumulation of life events and plays a role in the etiology of various somatic and psychiatric disorders Pileup as a way of looking at complex multiple role changes occurring within a short time period. This pile-up of changes may constitute a critical role transition and may provide a way to demarcate stages of family development Pile-up of family changes as the sum of normative and non-normative stressors and intrafamily strains, and provides one possible explanation for why some families may be more vulnerable to a single stressor or lack regenerative power or resiliency to recover from a crisis	71 items, each item in nine conceptual dimensions. Respondents check yes or no **Intrafamily strains**: two dimensions, 17 items; conflict—12 items that reflect sources of tension and conflict between family members. An increase in normative sources of intrafamily strain. Parenting strains—5 items related increased difficulties in enacting the parenting role **Marital strains**—4 items, measure stress in marital role arising from sexual or separation issues **Pregnancy & childbearing strains**—4 items, related to pregnancy difficulties or adding a new member **Finances & business strains**—12 items, two dimensions, family finances-9 items, assess sources of increased strains; Family business—3 tms reflect strains arising from a family qwned business **Work family transition & strains**—10 items; two dimensions, working transition—4 items related to moving in or out of the work force; family transition & work —6 items, focus on changes occurring at work or moved mad by the family **Illness & family care strains**-8 items: three dimensions, illness onset & child care—4 items dependent needs arising from injury or illness of a family member or friend; chronic ill—2 items increased difficultied; dependency strain—2 items, more help or care **Losses** –6 items; due to death or broken relationship **Transitions "in & out"** –5 items, reflect member moving back home or moving out **Family legal violations** – 5 items, focus on a member breaking society's law or mores

Instruments and Sources	Theory	Purpose/ Population/ Intention/ How did they come up with the concept	Dimensions / Concepts	Operationalization
Family Hardiness Index (FHI) 20 items, 4-point scale. McCubbin, M. A. McCubbin, H. I. Thompson, A. I. (1986, 1996)	Family stress	To measure family hardiness in resistance to stress. Developed to measure the characteristics of hardiness as a stress resistance and adaptation resource in families, which would function as a buffer or mediating factor in mitigating the effects of stressors and demands, and a facilitation of family adjustment and adaptation over time. FHI was developed to adapt the concept of individual hardiness to the family unit. FHI was guided by the concept of individual hardiness developed from the discipline of existential psychology by Kobasa. Research on hardiness in individuals has been conducted solely on males who were middle and upper level executives (Kobasa, 1979) and lawyers (Kobassa, 1982). A population of 304 nonclinical families was sampled as a part of the ongoing research of the family stress, coping and health project at the University of Wisconsin-Madison. Early FHI has four subscales: cooriented commitment, confidence, challenge, and control. Recently research has focused on three components: commitment, challenge, & control	Family hardiness / Family Resource, regenerative type **Hardiness** was shown to function as a resistance resource to buffer the effects of stressful life events and that had its greatest health preserving effect when stressful life events increased. **Family hardiness** specifically refers to the internal strengths and durability of the family units and is characterized by a sense of control over the outcomes of life events and hardships. Families view change as beneficial and growth producing, and have an active rather than passive orientation in adjusting to and managing stressful situations. **Commitment** implies a curiosity about life and a sense of meaningfulness of life **Challenge** reflects the belief that it is normal for life to change and that change brings about stimulation and growth rather than presenting a threat to security **Control** encompasses the belief that one can influence the course of events	20 items were constructed to fit three components of commitment, challenge, & control. Respondents assessed the degree (False, mostly false, mostly true, true) **Commitment**: 8 items, measure the family's sense of internal strengths, dependability and ability to work together. **Challenge**: 6 items, measure the family's efforts to be innovative, active, to experience new things and to learn. **Control**: 6 items, measure the family's sense of being in control of family life rather than being shaped by outside events and circumstances. High scores indicate greater levels of family hardiness.
Family Time and Routines Index (FTRI): 30 items, 4-point scale McCubbin, H. I. McCubbin, M. A. Thompson, A. I. (1986, 1996)	Family routine inventory	To measure family integration and stability. Developed to assess the type of activities and routines families use and maintain and the value they place upon these practices. Based on the family routines inventory developed by scholars (Jensen, James, Boyce, & Harnett, 1983) but was	Family time & routines / Family resources Family Bonding Family Coherence Family Celebration Quality of Family Life Adopt and practice are relatively reliable indices of family integration and stability which include effective ways of meeting	FTRI is a 32-items, consisting 8 subscales: **Parent-child togetherness**—5 items, measure the family's emphasis on establishing predictable communications between parent and children and adolescents; **Couple together**—4 items, measure the family's emphasis on establishing predictable routines to

Instruments and Sources	Theory	Purpose/ Population/ Intention/ How did they come up with the concept	Dimensions / Concepts	Operationalization
		modified and expanded upon to be more inclusive of other family life cycles stages, particularly the adolescent and launching stages which have a profound influence on family stability and continuity. Family units bridge generations, establish continuity in the present and in the midst of disruptions, and build a solid foundation of interpersonal supports needed to negotiate major transitions and transformations Assumed that family units develop routines and make time commitments around paired relationships, around family activities and practices, and around family system activities.	common problems and the ability to handle major crises. Family patterns of stability involving traditions, celebrations, and family routines, appear to be an essential part of family life.	promote communication between couples; **Child routines**—4 items, measure the family's emphasis on establishing predictable routines to promote child/teen's sense of autonomy and order; **Meal's together subscale**—2 items, measures the family's efforts to establish predictable routines to promote a meaningful connection with relatives; **Family time together**—4 items, measure the family's emphasis on family togetherness to include special events, caring, quiet time and family time; **Family chores routines**—2 items, measure the family's emphasis on establishing predictable routines to promote child and adolescent responsibilities in the home; **Relatives connection routines**—4 items; and **Family management routines**-5 items, measures the family's efforts to establish predictability needed to maintain family order in the home. Respondents assess the degree (0=False, 1=Mostly false, 2=Mostly true, and 3=True); the other score for the extent to which the routine is viewed value as important. For the importance scale, Not important=0, somewhat important=1, very important=2. Not applicable=0.
Family problem solving and coping (FPSC): 10 items with a four Likert scale McCubbin, M. A. McCubbin, H. I. Thompson, A. (1986, 1996)	Resiliency model of family stress, adjustment and adaptation	The index to assess the two dominants patterns in family communication, which appear to play an important part in family coping with hardships and life catastrophes. Developed specifically for family stress and resiliency research and to measure the problem solving and coping component in the resiliency	Family problem solving and coping Incendiary communication: is inflammatory in nature and tends to exacerbate a stressful situation. Affirming communication: Conveys support and caring and exerts a calming influence. Quality of family communication determines to a measurable degree how	10 items with 4-point Likert scale (0=false, 1=mostly false, 2=most true, 3=true); two five-item subscales: **Incendiary communication**: 5 items, is Positively associated with both employee and spouse appraisal of family system distress and negatively associated with family hardiness; is inflammatory in nature and tends to exacerbate a stressful

Instruments and Sources	Theory	Purpose/ Population/ Intention/ How did they come up with the concept	Dimensions / Concepts	Operationalization
		model. Adaptive coping strategies and problem solving communication patterns are more generalized ways of responding to family hardship and difficulties by creating a family environment or context of communication in which and through which family hardships and issues are addressed and resolved. A sample of 297 investment executive families who had recently experienced the market crisis; and a survey of 721 Wisconsin rural banking employees who had recently experienced the farm economy crisis.	families manage tension and strain and acquire a satisfactory level of family functioning, adjustment and adaptation.	situation: **Affirming communication**: 5 items, conveys support and caring and exerts a calming influence; was negatively associated with both employee and spouse appraisal of family system distress and positively associated with family hardiness. This subscale is a positive attribute.
Family Schema-Ethnic Index (FSCH-E): 39 items, 4-point Likert scale McCubbin, H. I. Thompson, A. Elver, K. Carpenter, K. (1992)	Family paradigm of function	Measure the degree to which a family has cultivated a family schema, a world view which is inclusive of cultural and ethnic values and which is an important part of the family's identity. Fostering family problem solving and coping, and its established patterns of functioning and family paradigm of functioning. Facilitates the development of meaning through the processes of classification, spiritualization, temporalization, and contextualization.	Family coherence / Family resource, Regenerative type Family schema/ Family identity, values, beliefs, rules, and boundaries. Family has cultivated a sense of cultural and ethnic values, which is an important part of the family's identity	39 items with 4-point Likert scale (0=False, 1=Mostly false, 2=mostly true, 3=true). Designed to record what are the core aspects of the family the degree to which the family has cultivated a sense of cultural and ethnic values. **Confidence** **Meaningfulness** **Manageability** **Comprehensibility**
Family Assessment Device (FAD): 53 items Epstein, N. B. Baldwin, L. B. Bishop, D. S. (1982)	McMaster Model of Family Functioning	To measure family functioning (problem solving, roles, affective responsiveness, affective involvement, behavior control, and general functioning). Designed to evaluate family functioning according to the McMaster model. Assume that family health is related to the accomplishment of essential functions and tasks.	Family adaptation / family funtioning Problem solving: family's ability to resolve problems. Communication: exchange of information among family members. Describe the outcome of family efforts to achieve a new level of balance and fit after a family crisis Defined as a minimal discrepancy between demands and capabilities at two primary	FAD assess 6 dimensions of family functioning **Problem solving** refers to the family's ability to resolve problems; **Communication**: is defined as the exchange of content and direct in the sense that the person spoken to is the person for whom the message is intended; **Roles** established patterns of behavior for handling a set of family

Instruments and Sources	Theory	Purpose/ Population/ Intention/ How did they come up with the concept	Dimensions / Concepts	Operationalization
		Developed on the basis of responses of 03 individuals of whom 294 came from a group of 112 families. The bulk of the families had one member who was an inpatient in an adult psychiatric hospital, 209 individuals were students in an introductory psychology course. Although the current version of the scale has 60 items, the original studies were based on a 53-item measure.	levels of interaction	functions which include provision of resources, providing nurturance and support, supporting personal development, maintaining and managing the family system and providing adult sexual gratification; **Affective Responsiveness** assesses the extent to which individual family members are able to experience appropriate affect over a range of stimuli; **Affective Involvement** is concerned with the extent to which family members are interested in and place value on each other's activities and concerns; **Behavioral control** assesses the way in which a family expresses and maintains standards of behavior of its members; **General Functioning**: evaluates family functioning. Each item is scored on a 1 to 4 basis using: 1=Strong agree, 2=Agree, 3=Disagree, 4=Strong disagree. Items describing unhealthy functioning are reverse-scored. Lower scores indicate healthier functioning. Scored responses to the items are averaged to provide seven scale scores, each having a possible range from 1 (healthy) to 4 (unhealthy).
Family Crisis Oriented Personal Evaluation Scales (F-COPES): 30 items, 5-point scale McCubbin, H. I. Olson, D. Larsen, A. (1981, 1996)	Resiliency model of family stress, adjustment and adaptation	To measure family coping F-COPES is to identify problem solving and behavioral strategies utilized by families in response to difficult or problematic situations. The items focus on the two levels of interaction outlined in the resiliency model. Individual relationship to family system and family to social environment. Designed to record effective problem-solving attitudes and behaviors which	Pile-up, Family coherence / Family resource and meaning/ perception The meaning a family attaches to a stressful situation, or the family's appraisal of the situation, may also serve as part of family's coping behavior. Coping behavior involves the management of various dimensions of family life simultaneously: maintaining satisfactory internal conditions for communication and family organization; promoting member independence and self-esteem; maintenance	30 items, five-point Likert scale (1=strongly disagree, 2=moderately disagree, 3= neither agree nor disagree, 4=moderately agree, 5=strongly agree): 8 subscales become 5 subscales. **Acquiring Social Support:** 9 items, measure a family's ability to actively engage in acquiring support from relatives, friends, neighbors and extended family; **Reframing:** 8 items, assesses the family's capability to redefine stressful events in order to make them more

Instruments and Sources	Theory	Purpose/ Population/ Intention/ How did they come up with the concept	Dimensions / Concepts	Operationalization
		families develop to respond to problems or difficulties. Based on the family stress theory, F-COPES was designed to integrate family resources and the meaning of perception factors into coping strategies. Factor analysis procedures were used to determine the underlying dimensions. A pilot study consisting of 49 items was constructed. A sample of 119 items was drawn from a university class with a combined population of undergraduate and graduate students. The eigenvalues were greater than one, and factor loading were greater than .38. The 49 items list was reduced to 30. Eight factors became to 5 factors.	and development of social supports in transactions with the community; and maintenance of some efforts to control the impact of the stressors and the amount of change in the family unit	manageable; **Seeking Spiritual Support:** 4 items, focus on the family's ability to acquire spiritual support; **Mobilizing Family to Acquire and Accept Help:** 4 items, measure the family's ability to seek out community resources and accept help from others; **Passive Appraisal:** 4 items, assess the family's ability to accept problematic issues minimizing reactivity.
Family Coping Coherence Index (FCCI): 4 items McCubbin, H. I. Larsen, A. Olson, D. (1982) manual@rmacc.wisc.edu Center for excellence in Family Studies, Family Stress, coping and health project	Sense of coherence	To measures family coherence and coping. Identify a subscale of family coping which related to concept of a sense of coherence which families call upon to manage life changes and stresses The FCCI emerged from the original F-COPES as a subscale, which measures the concept of coherence and its use as a coping tool for the family. Four items were selected which related to the constructs of manageability, control, trust, and confidence, which were defining concepts of the sense of coherence	Family coherence / Family resource, Regenerative type	Original: 71 items Family resource: Confidence in family problem solving, Reframing family problem. Family passivity; Social and community resource: church/ religious resource; extended families, friends, neighbors, community resources
Family Coping Coherence Index (Family Index of Regenerativity and Adaptation-Military: 17 items) McCubbin, H. I. & Patterson, J. M (1982)	Family Resources	Record the degree to which families call upon their appraisal skills to manage stressful life events, strains, and changes	Family coherence / Family resource, Regenerative type	Four-item with 5-point Likert scale ranging from strongly disagree to strongly agree. The index includes : acceptance of stressful events, accepting difficulties, a positive appraisal of a problem & having faith in God

Instruments and Sources	Theory	Purpose/ Population/ Intention/ How did they come up with the concept	Dimensions / Concepts	Operationalization
Family Index of regenerativity and adaptation-General (FIRA-G); McCubbin, H. I. (1987, 1996)	The Resiliency Model of Family Stress, Adjustment and Adaptation	FIRA-series is designed to obtain 7 indices of family functioning. Provide a brief set of measures, which have reliability and validity and can be used to test the major dimensions of the resiliency model. Use of self-report family systems assessment measure in research, education and clinical counseling work and particularly family health research is based on the premise that family processes interact with individual family members, but the research to substantiate this relationship is in an embryonic state of development. Guide family life education programs and family oriented clinical and health focused interventions, the training of family educators, nurses, social workers and physicians will continue to be guided by faith experience, clinical insights and unconfirmed assumptions. Address these educational and clinical issues about the families system, family assessment measures have been developed and tested. Facilitate research in the study of family systems, their transitions, family adjustment and adaptation, as well as their impact on family member. Made an effort to develop a cluster of family measures designed and selected to assess the critical dimensions and components of this family stress model. Three major survey of family strengths from 1036 military families, 1000 nonmilitary families and 304 nonmilitary families to compare 4-stages of the family cycle.	Family stressors/Pile-up Family strains/Pile-up Relative and friend support/Family support Social support/Community support Family coherence/ Family resources regenerative type Family hardiness/ Family resources regenerative type Family distress /Adaptation Family indices of regenerative and adaptation is a patterned after the resiliency model of family stress, adjustment, and adaptation, is designed to obtain reliable and valid indices of family stressors, family strains, relative and friend support, family confidence, family coherence, family hardiness and two indices of family adaptation-family discord and family distress. The concept of family adaptation is used to describe a continuum of outcomes that reflect family efforts to achieve a balance of functioning at the number-to-family and family-to-community levels. The positive end of the continuum called bonadaptaion	**Family stressors**: FILE (10 items) records life events and changes which can render a family vulnerable to the impact of a subsequent stressors or change. The index includes the addition of a member, changes in the work situation, deaths, and illness. **Family strains**: FILE (10 items) records life events and changes which can render a family vulnerable to the impact of a subsequent stressors or change. The index includes conflict between husband and wife, conflict among with children, financial hardships and the strains of caring for an ill member. **Relative and friend support**: FCOPES (8 items) support index records that families call upon support of relatives and friends as one of the strategies the family unit uses to mange its stressors and strains. **Social support**: SSI (17 items) records that families are integrated into the community, view the community as a source of support and feel that the community can provide emotional, self-esteem, and network support. **Family coherence**: FCOPES (4 items) records that families call upon their appraisal skills to manage stressful life events, strains, and changes including the acceptance of stressful events, accepting difficulties, a positive appraisal of a problem and having faith in God. **Family hardiness**: FHI (20 items) measure the characteristics of hardiness as a stress resistance and adaptation resources in families which would function as a buffer or mediating factor in mitigating the effects of stressors and

Instruments and Sources	Theory	Purpose/ Population/ Intention/ How did they come up with the concept	Dimensions / Concepts	Operationalization
				demands, and a facilitation of family adjustment and adaptation over time. **Family distress**: FILE (5 items) records the major difficulties families may experience which reflect a deterioration in a family's stability. The index includes family members with emotional problems, the abuse of alcohol or divorce and deterioration in the marital relationship Family stressor, Family strains and Damily distress scales: items answered yes=1 and no=0; the other 4 instruments (1=Strongly disagree, 2=disagree, 3=neutral, 4=agree, 5=strongly agree). Reversal (1=5, 2=4, 3=3, 4=2, 1=5) are needed for some of the items in the family hardiness and social support index in order to ensure all items were weighted in a positive direction for analysis and interpretation.

Family Functioning in Care for Children with Disabilities: Through Review

To bring an ill, handicapped, or disabled child into the world is one of the most heartbreaking events parents ever face. The disability experience affects the functioning of the whole family, as well as creating intense stress on the family and specifically on its total resources. Many studies evidenced that these families encountered enormous stressors (Longo & Bond, 1984). Longo and Bond (1984) integrated the impact of these stressors into four important areas: psychological well-being, the stability of the spouse relationship, the welfare of the siblings, and the overall family functioning.

Family function is one important aspect of caregivers' quality of life and is also affected by the disabled experience. The majority of the caregivers of the disabled children are parents or other family members. The disability experience affects the functioning of the whole family. The intense stress may result in disruption and break down of system functioning when the demands on the physical and psychological energy or other resources are too great. The chronic stress leads families to utilize many coping mechanisms to change internal and external conditions. Families experience growth and integration, balance and stability, and disorder and disintegration (Bubolz & Whiren, 1984). Many studies evidence exists that these families encountered enormous stressors (Longo & Bond, 1984). Longo and Bond (1984) integrated the impact of these stressors into four important areas: psychological well-being, the stability of the spouse relationship, the welfare of siblings and overall family functioning.

From the studies reviewed, it is clear that family functioning as it relates to families has a number of aspects. These aspects include problem solving, communication, role, international relationship, organization system, and affective responsiveness. Many now are proposed to evaluate the family's impact on health (Halvorsen, 1991; Koranek, 1989). However, the concept of family functioning has not been defined systematically within a theoretical framework. There is disagreement on key concepts and definition of family functioning. Little examined the family as a functioning micro system of society making adaptation in a complex social environment.

The aims of this article are to identify the concept of the family functioning, and related theory. The other is to provide a psychometric critique of family functioning instruments that have been used with families of disabled children.

Method

Procedure

A system review of research of the literature using MEDLINE (1990-2003) and CINAHL (1990-2003) databases located studies that focused on the family functioning of children with a disability or handicapped. The keywords used in the search were handicapped or disability child and family functioning. The search yielded a total of 26 citations. An examination of the citations indicated that three family functioning instruments had been used in research with families of children with handicapped or a disability: Family Assessment Device (FAD), Family APGAR (FAPGAR), and Family Environment Scale (FES).

Articles detailing the psychometric properties of the identified quality of life instruments were located by searching MEDLINE (1990 –2003) and CINAHL (1990 –2003) databases using the name of the instrument and instrument research, and psychometric properties as keywords. A total of 35 articles were located.

Concept of Family Functioning

The family is a complex system of interacting individuals. McGoldrick and Carter (2003) referred that "families consist of persons who have a shared history and a shared future (p. 376)." Families also have roles and functions. Family functioning may be defined in terms of process, outcome, or content (Robert & Feetham, 1983). Family functioning is more related to transactional and systemic properties of the family system. It includes providing nurturance and support, maintaining, and managing the family system. The basic attributes of family functioning are characterized and explained how a family system typically appraises, operates, and behaves (McCubbin & Thompson, 1991). Different models of family functioning explain different dimensions or attributes of family functioning.

Smith (1995) identified structure as "the number of members of the family and to the designation of familial positions such as parents, spouse, child, other kin, etc. (p.9)", and referred function to manners as families satisfy members' physical and psychological needs and to meet survival and maintenance needs (p. 9)." Shek (1999) suggested understanding family by three levels: the functioning of individual family members, the functioning of dyadic relationship (husband-wife dyad and parent-child dyad), and the functioning of the whole family (family competence, family coherence, family atmosphere).

Family functioning is a set of basic attributes about family system that characterize and explain how a family system appraises, operates, and behaves (McCubbin & McCubbin,

1991). Family functioning can be found to solve problems, to present affection, to play the major role, and to meet the families' needs. The ability to maintain a balance between change and stability has been referred to as one nature of healthy family functioning (Olson, 1993). Family functioning was a reliable predictor of parent adjustment.

Healthy family functioning does not refer to an absence of problems (Walsh, 2003). Walsh (2003) emphasize that "the healthy family can be found in the midst problems as in family resilience (p. 5)." Minuchin (1974) has advocated that no families are problem-free. Therefore, the presence of distress is not necessarily a criterion of family pathology, and healthy family functioning depends on the fit or compatibility among individuals, family, social, and cultural systems (Walsh, 2003).

Models of Family Functioning

The McMaster Model of Family Functioning comprises six dimensions: problem solving, communication, roles, affective responsiveness, affective involvement, and behavioral control (Epstein, Baldwin, & Bishop, 1982). The McMaster model is a view of healthy family functioning (Epstein, Bishop, Ryan, Miller, & Keitner, 2003). Epstein et al. (2003) identified "family problem solving as a family ability to resolve problems to a level that maintains effective family functioning (p. 587), communication as the exchange of verbal information within a family (p. 589), family role as the repetitive patterns of behavior by which family members fulfill family functions (p. 590), affective responsiveness as the ability to respond to a given stimulus with an appropriate quality and quantity of feelings (p. 594), behavior control as the pattern a family adopts for handling behavior in three areas— physically dangerous situations, involving meeting and expressing psychobiological needs and drives, and interpersonal socializing behavior (p. 596)."

The Circumplex model of family functioning (Couple and Family Map) related to three major components: family cohesion, flexibility (adaptability), and communication (Olson, Sprenkle, & Russell, 1979; Olson & Gorall, 2003). The family Adaptability and Cohesion Evaluation Scale (FACES) based on the Model designed to assess family type. Olson and Gorall (2003) identified "family cohesion as the emotional bonding that couple and family members have toward one another (p. 516), family flexibility (family adaptability) as the mount of change in its leadership, role relationship, and relationship rules (p.519), communication as a critical for facilitating couples and families to alter their levels of cohesion and flexibility (p. 520)." Within the model there are five levels of cohesion ranging from disengaged/disconnected, to somewhat connected, to connected, to very connected, to overly connected (enmeshed). The five levels of flexibility range from rigid/inflexible to somewhat flexible, to flexible, to very flexible, to chaotic/overly flexible (Olson & Gorall, 2003).

The Beavers System Model has two dimensions of family functioning: competence and style (Beavers & Hampson, 2003). Competence refers to how well families perform the skills to deal with the tensions between individual choice and group needs and between the need for individual freedom and the need for belonging and togetherness, to negotiate and share leadership, and to establish strength. Five classifications of families range from optimal, to adequate, to midrange, to borderline, severely dysfunctional (Beavers & Hampson, 2003). Family style is the family members' patterns of interaction and orientation to receiving gratification. Three types of family style are tripetal, mixed, and centrifugal (Beavers & Hampson, 2003). The more competent the family, the more balanced and flexible is the family style, which enables members to adapt (Beavers & Hampson, 2003).

Dimensions of above three models are related to family process. Each model reflects the values and beliefs of the theorist who develop it. In addition, the social-ecological-psychological and system theory was utilized to develop the Family Environment Scale (FES). The basic unit of analysis of the ecological model is microsystem that is the immediate perceived environment of the person (individual's personality characteristics on family interactions). The next level is the mesosystem that connects between multiple microsystems (effects of spousal relationships on parent-child interactions). Microsystems and mesosystems are embedded within exosystems, which are settings that have indirect effects on family interactions (effects of a parent's work patterns on relationships among family members). The macrosystem is overarching economic, political, cultural, and social forces that influence individuals (effect of social and economic class on family functioning) (Meyers, Varkey, & Aguirre, 2002).

The FES had three major dimensions: Interpersonal relationship, growth, and system maintenance (Moos & Moos, 1981). The dimension of the model is related to family context. Communications and relationships are the extent to which family members feel they belong to, are involved with, and are supportive of one another; the extent of open expression of emotion among family members; and the amount of conflictual interaction in the family environment. Personal growth assesses the amount of independence that individuals may attain within the system and their personal orientation in various areas. System maintenance reflects the degree of structure, clarity of rules, and openness to change that characterizes the family; the extent to which order and organization are important; the degree to which rules and authority are maintained in the family system; and the ability of the family to regulate emotional boundaries (Peleg-Popko & Klingman, 2002). The FES was applied to measure global family functioning and environment that include assessing cohesion, expressiveness, conflict, independence, achievement, knowledge, entertainment, moral/religious belief, organization, and control (Moos & Moos, 1986).

The resiliency model assists nursing professionals assessing family functioning and intervening in a family system to promote family adjustment, and family adaptation, as well as determining what family types, capabilities, and strengths are needed. In addition, the model also is designed to help the professional create strategies for intervention based on evaluation of the family functioning under stress (McCubbin & McCubbin, 1993). The other specific concepts used to describe healthy family functioning and unhealthy family functioning are different from these conceptual models.

Family Functioning of Care of a Disabled Child

Disabled child and family functioning were studies in patients with various diagnoses, mental retardation, depression (Fornari et al., 1999; Stein et al., 2000; Tamplin & Goodyer, 2001; Tamplin, Goodyer, & Herbert, 1998), psychiatric disorders (Friedmann et al., 1997), traumatic brain injury (Rivara et al., 1996b), down syndrome, physical disability (Luescher, Dede, Gitten, Fennell, & Maria, 1999), epilepsy (Magill-Evans, Darrah, Pain, Adkins, & Kratochvil, 2001; Pal, Chaudhury, Das, & Sengupta, 2002), DMD (Reid & Renwick, 2001), developmental disability (Lobato & Kao, 2002), mental retardation (Costigan, Floyd, Harter, & McClintock), cerebral palsy, spinal bifida, and hydrocephalus (King, King, Rosenbaum, & Goffin, 1999), suicide (King, Segal, Naylor, & Evans, 1993), fracture (Loder, Warschausky, Schwartz, Hensinger, & Greenfield, 1995), and anorexia nervosa (Gowers & North, 1999). The result of these studies indicated a relationship between family functioning and the disabled.

Summarizing the studies, all included a conceptual model or theory of family functioning. Most of these studies used the Family Assessment Device to explore family function and its related effects.

Family Resources

Family support and family communication promote hardiness in families with a disabled child. Parent-child bonding managed well that can increase positive dynamic and maintain effective communication, obtain family hardiness and coherence.

Family Support. Olsen, Marshall, Mandleco, Allred, Dyches, and Sansom (1999) examined how family support and perceptions of family incendiary communication (N=54 set of parents with disabled children) were related to hardiness in families with disabled children including speech disorders, developmental delays, down syndrome, and mental retardation.

Parental Bonding. Stein et al. (2000) evaluated parent-child bonding (using Parental Bonding Instrument, PBI) and family functioning (using the Family Assessment Device, FAD) in depressed children (N=54), children at high risk for depression (N=21), and low-risk controls (N=23). The result found that maternal depression effect on the child's perception of maternal protection and paternal care, mother's report on all FAD scales, and father's report on most FAD scales. The child with major depressive disorder reported significantly lower on the FAD scales of behavioral control and general functioning of the father's scores. Mothers of high-risk children had significantly lower scores on the roles and affective involvement of the FAD compared with the mothers of low-risk children.

Family Hardiness and Coherence. Failla et al., (1991) addressed the interaction of key components that affect family functioning in a study with 57 mothers of children with developmental disability. Results indicated positive relationships between family hardiness, coherence, and functional support, and satisfaction with family function. The study suggests that family hardiness could diminish the effects of stress, increase the use of support, and facilitate adaptation.

Social Support. Pal, Chaudhury, Das, and Sengupta (2002) tested the hypothesis that maternal satisfaction with social support, measured 46 mothers of children aged 6-18 years with epilepsy at the beginning of treatment, would predict parental adjustment to the child's epilepsy after 1 year of treatment. They measured social support using the modified Dunst family support scale, and parental adjustment using a locally validated instrument. Parental adjustment at outcome was positively independently correlated with satisfaction with social support at baseline, and negatively with severity of the child's epilepsy.

Magill-Evans, Darrah, Pain, Adkins, and Kratochvil (2001) compared adolescents with cerebral palsy (CP) and their families to adolescents without physical disabilities and their families as the child enters and leaves adolescence (age ranges 13 to 15 years and 19 to 23 years). Families of 90 individuals with CP (42 females, 48 males) and 75 individuals without physical disabilities (34 females, 41 males) participated. There were few differences in family functioning, life satisfaction, or perceived social support between the groups. Expectations of young adults with CP and parents of both adolescents and young adults regarding future independence and success were lower than the expectations of the control group.

Service Needs

Caretaking demands were at risk for added stress in social, isolation, and reduced autonomy. The families must deal with maladaptation or unhealthy dynamic. Poor problem solving, communication, and role allocation, and social leisure problem often existed in disabled children with families with depression.

Hendriks, De Moor, Oud, and Franken (2000) described service needs of eighty-four families' parents of toddlers with motor or multiple disabilities. The results indicated the family needs understanding the child's disability, information on community services, and help in parenting. Mothers feel more need than fathers for support and for help in explaining their child's condition to others. Help in family functioning did not include in the factor analysis for this group. Initially, the family must deal with the child's most urgent needs. Then the family requests more assistance for their own functioning and environmental demands.

Functioning

Max, et al. (1997) assessed prospectively the risk factor related to the onset of a novel psychiatric disorder in the first three months after traumatic brain injury in children aged 6 to 14 years. They found that family function was one of the significant predictors of novel psychiatric disorder.

Rivara, Jaffe, Polissar, Fay, Liao, and Martin (1996) examined changes in family functioning from injury to 3 years after pediatric traumatic brain injury in families of 81 children; to determine factors most predictive of family outcomes at 3 years and variables that promote positive outcomes and changes over time. Preinjury functioning was the best predictor of 3-year outcomes. Fewer changes in family functioning were reported over 3 years in the mild or moderate groups, whereas more deterioration occurred in the severe group. Better preinjury levels of communication, expressiveness, problem solving, use of resources, role flexibility, greater activity orientation, and less conflict, control, and stress marked positive change for the severe group.

The families of patients with schizophrenic disorders, major depression, bipolar disorder, substance abuse, and adjustment disorders reported poor family functioning compared to control families in the areas of problem solving, communication, roles, affective responsiveness, affective involvement, and general functioning. Families of patients with anxiety disorders reported poor problem solving, communication, and general functioning than nonclinical families, the families of patients with eating disorders reported only poor problem solving and communication compared to control families (Friedmann et al., 1997). A higher proportion of families in the subjects except the families of patients with eating disorders reported unhealthy communication within the family compared to control families. A higher proportion of schizophrenic spectrum, depressed, and bipolar patient families fell in the unhealthy affective responsiveness compared to control families. Compared to nonclinical families, unhealthy role functioning was reported by a larger proportion of families in all psychiatric groups except for eating and anxiety disorders (Friedmann et al., 1997). The findings presented that the families of psychiatric patients experience higher levels of dysfunction compared to nonclinical families. Having a family member in the acute phase of a psychiatric disorder appears to be a risk factor for poor family functioning across many areas, including problem solving, communication, affect expression and responsiveness, role allocation, and general functioning (Friedmann et al., 1997).

King, Segal, Naylor, and Evans (1993) identified family and parental characteristics associated with suicidal behavior among adolescent inpatients with mood disorders. They used three groups—32 suicidal adolescent inpatients with mood disorders, 32 nonsuicidal adolescent inpatients with mood disorders, and 38 normal comparison adolescents to compare with the Family Assessment Device Score, Hamilton Rating Scale for Depression, and Social Adjustment Scale-Self Report Score. And the parents measures were the Symptom Checklist-90 and the Social Adjustment Scale-Self Report. The suicidal group stated that their families were most dysfunctional and least affectively responsive; and the depression severity was related to negative perceptions of family functioning. The suicidal adolescents' fathers reported more family unit adjustment problems than did both nonsuicidal and normal comparison adolescents' father. Suicidal mothers reported more family unit and social/leisure problems than did normal comparison group mothers. The study evidenced that a maladaptive or unhealthy dynamic within the families of suicidal adolescents with mood disorders.

Reid and Renwick (2001) investigated 36 caregivers and 32 adolescents and the relationships between familial stress and psychosocial adjustment in adolescents with DMD. The adolescents demonstrate lower levels of psychosocial adjustment than their normal reference group. The results also indicate that familial stress is associated with psychosocial adjustment in the adolescent and with intellectual function of the adolescent ($P = 0.001$).

Problem Solving. Costigan, Floyd, Harter, and McClintock (1997) examined family problem-solving interactions in families (N=165) of school-aged children with mild or moderate mental retardation and comparison sample (N=52). The results found that a disruptive impact of children with mental retardation in the form of more directiveness by mothers and fathers, less supportive problem solving by single mothers, and less active problem solving by the target children in the mental retardation group. The mothers engaged in relatively more supportive problem solving than fathers and they displayed more active listening than the fathers. The children with mental retardation had difficulty with the problem-solving task and engaged in less active problem solving than the comparison group. And the girls with mental retardation revealed fewer disruptive, negative behaviors than the comparison girls.

Emotional and Behavior Control. King, King, Rosenbaum, and Goffin (1999) examined the strength of the relationship between parents' perceptions of family-centered, professionally provided caregiving and their emotional well-being by using 164 parents of children with nonprogressive neurodevelopmental disorders (cerebral palsy, spina bifida, or hydrocephalus). The results showed that more family centered caregiving was a significant predictor of parents' well-being. Child behavior problems and protective factors in the social environment (family functioning and social support) are the most important predictors of well-being.

Intervention Program

Lobato and Kao (2002) evaluated an integrated group intervention for siblings (N=54) and parents designed to increase sibling understanding of and adjustment to chronic illness and developmental disability. The results showed that sibling knowledge of the child's disorders and sibling connectedness increased, and sibling reports of negative adjustment to the disorder and parent reports of sibling global behavioral functioning decreased significantly from pre- to post-treatment for the subjects. And parent satisfaction with the program was high.

Critique of the Body of Literature

The research on family functioning of disabled children is very limited especially for the motor disability with genetic problem. The products of empirics include describing, explaining, predicting, and intervention; it involves the scientific method of inquiry. It has usually been a subcategory of studies in a field of specific care, which focused on care of psychological problems, mental retardation, epilepsy, and developmental disability. The samples were usually not generalized to include all families with special problems with disabled children.

There was very little information from a cultural perspective exploring the experiences of family functioning. Most of the studies have been quantitative to identify the dimensions of the family functioning and to predict the risk factors related to the family functioning. In quantitative researches, the researchers identified the selected variables to be explored. Family support, parent-child bonding, family hardiness and coherence, social support, communication, behavioral control, expression, affective involvement, problem solving, and comorbid are dimensions found in the family functioning and are reflected in the professional code of conduct. Relevant to the concept of family functioning is the concept of dysfunction, unhealthy dynamics, and healthy functioning. Dysfunctional families are least affective responsive, more having social leisure problems, isolation, poor problem solving and communication. Families with depression are negative perception of family functioning and have family unit adjustment problem, maladaptation, or unhealthy dynamic. The majority of the family resources are family support and communication. Therefore, there is insufficient information to draw a complete model in order to interpret the family functioning.

Two studies presenting longitudinal data showed that family functioning was the best predictor of family outcome and psychiatric disorder. Better family functioning (including effective communication, expressiveness, problem solving, use of resources and role flexibility), less conflict, and more behavior control are stress marked positive change. Anxious, depressed, and suicidal families reported poor problem solving, communication, and general functioning. There are different behaviors and perceptions of family functioning in gender. Mothers are more supportive problem solvers, affective involvement, and active listeners. In addition, single mothers are less supportive problem solvers and are less aggressive about solving problems.

Eleven studies presented in the literature show cross-sectional data concerning family functioning, parent-child bonding, problem solving interactions, emotional well-being, and relationship. Results showed family functioning are not always negative nor always positive. In schizophrenic families, and families with severe mental retardation support the impact of family functioning. Some studies findings indicated that disabled families get family support and family resources to promote hardiness in families with a disabled child.

Gap in the literature

Analysis of the preceding studies indicates that the influence of family functioning on disabled families, both in longitudinal, and cross-sectional data, has mixed results and lack of support for the influence factors of family functioning on a disabled child. Several studies support families with psychological problems that scores of family functioning were lower than the control group. Other disabled families have not revealed similar results.

Direction for Research

The phenomenon of family functioning is a dynamic process and complex environment. The measurement of family functioning using quantitative inquiry might have limitations in expressing families' feelings. It is also difficult to understand the families' psychological changes during the disabled process. Exploring family function should consider the cultural background of the families. There are a lot of issues and influence factors cannot be clarified; it is hard to establish a theoretical model of family functioning for families with a disabled child. Thus, the research direction might need to shift to a structural equation model and qualitative approach to discover and conceptualize the complex interaction process.

Conclusion

The disability of the DMD child induces the family to change and influences the entire family system (Botvin, Radford, & Neumann, 1984; Siegel, Davidson, Kornfeld, & McCready, 1983). Family structure, process, and functioning are used to meet the demands for change in family relationships, activities and goals in the families. Families also play the role of a change mediator that places an emphasis on positive family functioning (Epstein, Bishop, Ryan, Miller, & Keitner, 1993).

Having a child with disabled child places enormous burdens upon how families function. The families experienced many challenges over their life that made them at risk and used their ability to maintain healthy functioning. Many studies evidenced these families had innumerable stressors. The impact of these stressors on adaptation and function in four major areas: psychological well-being of the parents, the stability of the spousal relationship, the welfare of the siblings and overall family functioning (Longo & Bond, 1984). When the families are able to create their strength and abilities, they are more resilient to the stress and challenges and they minimize negative outcomes. In the resilient family we can find the family that adapts to stress leads to higher level of functioning.

When a family experiences an illness-induced family stress—having a child with disability—the accumulated stress is the consequences of family efforts to cope and intrafamily and social ambiguity. Family types and patterns of functioning develop on the basis of family strengths and predict family adaptation (McCubbin & McCubbin, 1993). Several types and patterns of functioning were noted to emphasize different aspects of family functioning. The family strengths point to the importance of family attributes and patterns that emphasized family integrity, unity, flexibility, and predictability to manage the illness and its hardships (McCubbin & McCubbin, 1993). However, a stressor as powerful as the severity of disability of a disabled child produces a pile-up of demands and the family becomes increasing vulnerable.

Parent's and child's depression influence the parent-child bonding and family functioning in depressed and at risk. The professionals need early and prompt treatment of families' depression that should improve parent-child relations and family functioning.

References

Beavers, W. R., & Hampson, R. B. (2003). Measuring family competence: The Beavers
    System Model. In F. Walsh (Ed.), *Normal family process*. New York: Guilford.

Botvin, M. J. G., Radford, L. M., & Neumann, E. M. (1984). Psychosocial aspects of death
    and dying in Duchenne muscular dystrophy. *Archieve of Physical Medical
    Rehabilitation, 65*(79-82).

Bubolz, M. M., & Whiren, A. P. (1984). The family of the handicapped: An ecological model
    for policy and practice. *Family Relations, 33*(5-12).

Costigan, C. L., Floyd, F. J., Harter, K. S. M., & McClintock, J. C. (1997). Family process
    and adaptation to children with mental retardation: Disruption and resilience in family
    problem-solving interactions. *Journal of Family Psychology December, 11*(4), 515-
    529.

Epstein, N. B., Baldwin, L. B., & Bishop, D. S. (1982). McMaster Family Assessment Device,
    Version 3. In C. I. Carlson (Ed.), *Family assessment: A guide to methods and
    measures.* (pp. 340-343). New York: Guilford.

Epstein, N. B., Bishop, D. S., Ryan, C. E., Miller, I. W., & Keitner, G. I. (1993). The
    McMaster Model: View of healthy family functioning. In F. Walsh (Ed.), *Normal
    family processes* (pp. 138-160). New York: Guilford.

Epstein, N. B., Bishop, D. S., Ryan, C. E., Miller, I. W., & Keitner, G. I. (2003). The
    McMaster Model: View of healthy family functioning. In F. Walsh (Ed.), *Normal
    family processes* (3 ed., pp. 581-607). New York: Guilford.

Fornari, V., Wlodarczyk-Bisaga, K., Matthews, M., Sandberg, D., Mandel, F. S., & Katz, J. L.
    (1999). Perception of family functioning and depressive symptomatology in
    individuals with anorexia nervosa or bulimia nervosa. *Comprehensive Psychiatry.,
    40*(6), 434-441.

Friedmann, M. S., McDermut, W. H., Solomon, D. A., Ryan, C. E., Keitner, G. I., & Miller, I.
    W. (1997). Family functioning and mental illness: a comparison of psychiatric and
    nonclinical families.[comment]. *Family Process., 36*(4), 357-367.

Gowers, S., & North, C. (1999). Difficulties in family functioning and adolescent anorexia
    nervosa.[comment]. *British Journal of Psychiatry., 174*, 63-66.

Halvorsen, J. G. (1991). Self-report family assessment instruments: An evaluative review.
    Family Practice Research Journal, 11(1), 21-55.

Hendriks, H. C., De Moor, M. H., Oud, H. L., & Franken, W. M. (2000). Service needs of parents with motor or multiply disabled children in Dutch therapeutic toddler classes. *Clinical Rehabilitation, 14*, 506-517.

King, C. A., Segal, H. G., Naylor, M., & Evans, T. (1993). Family functioning and suicidal behavior in adolescent inpatients with mood disorders. *Journal of the American Academy of Child & Adolescent Psychiatry., 32*(6), 1198-1206.

King, G., King, S., Rosenbaum, P., & Goffin, R. (1999). Family-centered caregiving and well-being of parents of children with disabilities: linking process with outcome. *Journal of Pediatric Psychology, 24*(1), 41-53.

Koranek, M. F. a. A. g. t. m. a. m. (1989). Self-report measures of whole-family functioning. In H. D. Grotevant & I. Carlson (Eds.), *Family assessment: A guide to methods and measures* (pp. 66-108). New York: Guilford.

Lobato, D., & Kao, B. T. (2002). Integrated sibling-parent group intervention to improve sibling knowledge and adjustment to chronic illness and disability. *Journal of Pediatric Psychology, 27*(8), 711-716.

Loder, R. T., Warschausky, S., Schwartz, E. M., Hensinger, R. N., & Greenfield, M. L. (1995). The psychosocial characteristics of children with fractures. *Journal of Pediatric Orthopedics., 15*(1), 41-46.

Longo, D. C., & Bond, L. (1984). Families of the handicapped child: Research and practice. *Family Relations, 33*, 57-65.

Luescher, J. L., Dede, D. E., Gitten, J. C., Fennell, E., & Maria, B. L. (1999). Parental burden, coping, and family functioning in primary caregivers of children with Joubert syndrome. *Journal of Child Neurology., 14*(10), 642-648; discussion 669-672.

Magill-Evans, J., Darrah, J., Pain, K., Adkins, R., & Kratochvil, M. (2001). Are families with adolescents and young adults with cerebral palsy the same as other families? *Developmental Medicine & Child Neurology, 43*(7), 466-472.

Max, J. E., Smith, W. L. J., Sato, Y., Mattheis, P. J., Castillo, C. S., Lindgren, S. D., Robin, D. A., & Stierwalt, J. (1997). Traumatic brain injury in children and adolescents: Psychiatric disorders in the first three months. *Journal of the American Academy of child & Adolescent Psychiatry, 36*(1), 94-102.

McCubbin, H. I., & Thompson, A. I. (1991). *Family assessment inventories for reseach and practice*. Madison: University of Wisconsin.

McCubbin, M. A., & McCubbin, H. I. (1991). Family stress theory and assessment: The resiliency model of family stress, adjustment, and adpatation. In A. I. Thompson (Ed.), *Family assessment inventories for research and practice* (pp. 3-34). Madison: University of Wisconsin.

McCubbin, M. A., & McCubbin, H. I. (1993). Families coping with illness: The resiliency model of family stress, adjustment, and adaptation. In P. Winstead-Fry (Ed.), *Families, health, & illness: Perspectives on coping and intervention* (pp. 21-63). St. Louis: Mosby.

McGoldrick, M., & Carter, B. (2003). The family life cycle. In F. Walsh (Ed.), *Normal family process* (3 ed., pp. 375-398). New York: Guilford.

Meyers, S. A., Varkey, S., & Aguirre, A. M. (2002). Ecological correlates of family functioning. *American Journal of Family Therapy, 30*, 257-273.

Moos, R. H., & Moos, B. S. (1981). *Family Environment Scale Manual*. Palo Alto, CA: Consulting Psychologists.

Moos, R. H., & Moos, B. S. (1986). *Environment Scale Manual*. Palo Alto, CA: Consulting Psychologists.

Olsen, S. F., Marshall, E. S., Mandleco, B. L., Allred, K. W., Dyches, T. T., & Sansom, N. S. (1999). Support, communication, and Hardiness in families with children with disabilites. *1999, 5*(3), 275-291.

Olson, D., Sprenkle, D., & Russell, C. (1979). Circumplex model of marital and family systems: I. Cohesion and adaptability dimensions, family types and clinical applications. *Family Process, 18*, 3-28.

Olson, D. H. (1993). Circumplex model of marital and family systems: Assessinf family functioning. In F. Walsh (Ed.), *Normal family processes*. New York: Guildford.

Olson, D. H., & Gorall, D. M. (2003). Circumplex model of marital and family systems. In F. Walsh (Ed.), *Normal family processes:Growing diversity and complexity*. New York: Guilford.

Pal, D. K., Chaudhury, G., Das, T., & Sengupta, S. (2002). Predictors of parental adjustment to children's epilepsy in rural India. *Child: Care, Health & Development, 28*(4), 295-300.

Peleg-Popko, O., & Klingman, A. (2002). Family environment, discrepancies between perceived actual and desirable environment and children's test and trait anxiety. *British Journal of Guidance and Counselling, 30*, 451-466.

Reid, D. T., & Renwick, R. M. (2001). Relating familial stress to the psychosocial adjustment of adolescents with Duchenne muscular dystrophy. *International Journal of Rehabilitation Research, 24*(2), 83-93.

Rivara, J. M., Jaffe, K. M., Polissar, N. L., Fay, G. C., Liao, S., & Martin, K. M. (1996a). Predictors of family functioning and change 3 years after traumatic brain injury in children. *Archives of Physical Medicine & Rehabilitation, 77*(8), 754-764.

Rivara, J. M., Jaffe, K. M., Polissar, N. L., Fay, G. C., Liao, S., & Martin, K. M. (1996b). Predictors of family functioning and change 3 years after traumatic brain injury in children.[comment]. *Archives of Physical Medicine & Rehabilitation., 77*(8), 754-764.

Robert, C. S., & Feetham, S. L. (1983). Assessing family functioning across three areas of relationships. *Nursing Research, 31*, 231-235.

Siegel, I. M., Davidson, H., Kornfeld, M., & McCready, W. C. (1983). Coping with muscular dystrophy: Psychosocial correlates of adaptation. *Muscle and Nerve, 6*, 607-609.

Stein, D., Williamson, D. E., Birmaher, B., Brent, D. A., Kaufman, J., Dahl, R. E., Perel, J. M., & Ryan, N. D. (2000). Parent-child bonding and family functioning in depressed children and children at high risk and low risk for future depression. *Journal of the American Academy of Child & Adolescent Psychiatry., 39*(11), 1387-1395.

Tamplin, A., & Goodyer, I. M. (2001). Family functioning in adolescents at high and low risk for major depressive disorder. *European Child & Adolescent Psychiatry., 10*(3), 170-179.

Tamplin, A., Goodyer, I. M., & Herbert, J. (1998). Family functioning and parent general health in families of adolescents with major depressive disorder. *Journal of Affective Disorders., 48*(1), 1-13.

Walsh, F. (2003). Changing families in a changing world: Reconstructing family normality. In F. Walsh (Ed.), *Normal family processes* (3 ed., pp. 3-26). New York: Guilford.

Part Five

Applied, Generated and Disseminated

Functioning among Taiwanese Families with a Child

Having Duchenne Muscular Dystrophy

INTRODUCTION

Overview

Little is understood about how Taiwanese families function when they have a child with Duchenne Muscular Dystrophy (DMD). Resilience, as well as hardiness, are important qualities found in families coping with other life stressors, and may also be factors in how DMD families function. The sacrifices families must make when a child has DMD - related disabilities are not temporary. Instead they become a way of life for the whole family and often require services from many agencies, which may result in increased financial costs, social isolation, as well as restriction of life-styles and career opportunities (Failla & Jones, 1991; Gottlieb, 1998; Patterson & McCubbin, 1983). The reciprocal impacts on the families are circular and continuous (Patterson, 2002).

Background and Significance

DMD, the second most common genetic disease in humans, is an X-linked disease of the muscle caused by mutation of the Xp21 gene. This gene encodes a rod like cytoskeletal protein called dystrophin that afflicts only boys who inherit the disease from their mothers (Emery, 1993; Nicholson, 1993). The world wide incidence, based on live male births, is around 200 to 300 x 10^{-6}, but the mutation rate is approximately 70 to 100 x 10^{-6} (Emery, 1993; Laing, 1993).

As children get older, DMD takes a slow and arduous course that leads to parental strains. The children's emotional responses in the form of problem behavior resulting from social isolation and poor interpersonal skills, has been found to predict maternal stress and anxiety (Huang & Dai, 1998; Nereo, Fee, & Hinton, 2003; Nereo & Hinton, 2003).

The progression of the children's disabilities induces the family to change and influences the entire family system (Botvin, Radford, & Neumann, 1984; Siegel, Davidson, Kornfeld, & McCready, 1983). Family structure, process, and functioning change the most as a result of the demands on family relationships, activities, and goals of the family social system (Thompson, Zeman, Fanurik, & Sirotkin-Roses, 1992). Families also change roles to meet the demands for achieving positive family functioning (Epstein, Bishop, Ryan, Miller, & Keitner, 1993). Some families adapt and others become depleted of family energy and resources; this difference has received little attention in the pediatric literature (Thompson et al., 1992).

The theoretical and empirical basis of a family-oriented approach has not been widely addressed, even in Taiwan, limiting the efforts of family health and human service providers involved in family health promotion. Health professionals have the responsibility to strengthen the family/child's coping resources and make the children's environment more accommodating to their special needs, as well as to assist their families to enrich their lives through interventions that enhance meaning and satisfaction in caregiving through positive experience and encounters.

The ability to maintain a balance between change and stability has been referred to as a measure of healthy family functioning. When families are able to utilize their strength and abilities, they are able to recover from the stress and challenge and minimize a negative outcome. The resilient family that adapts to stress has a higher level of functioning. Families that function well can solve problems, share affection, and meet the needs of individual family members.

If nursing professionals could evaluate family resilience and discuss interventions to support it, they could promote family functioning. And if the family of a DMD child can describe how they have dealt with the disability and anticipated loss, this might help others in similar situations to deal with their own sense of loss, fatigue, and distress. This study attempts to discover which family characteristics, supports, strengths, resources, and functioning buffer the impact of a stressful life and improve understanding of why some families thrives and other families do not. The findings of this study may contribute to the development of interventions that will help promote resilience in family members living with a child having DMD.

Statement of the Problem

The progressive disabling condition of DMD creates disruptions in the physical, social, emotional, and spiritual life of the affected child and his family. The chronic stress experienced by these families challenges their coping mechanisms as they adjust and continue to function. Families may experience growth and integration, balance and stability, or disorder and disintegration (Bubolz & Whiren, 1984). For family members, a DMD diagnosis heralds deformity with immobility, creating the need for important social services, such as special education programs, respite programs, and insurance coverage. DMD challenges a family to maintain normal functioning while struggling with loss.

The philosophy and policy trends of normalization and de-institutionalization encourage families to raise children with developmental disabilities at home. As more disabled children stay at home, families must become more diverse in their skills to meet the challenges and special risks that accompany a DMD diagnosis. In addition, the ability of these families to function at this level must also be viewed in light of a Taiwanese society which is evolving into one that is increasingly multiracial, multicultural, and multilingual (Braverman, 2001; Wisensale, 1993).

Analysis of longitudinal and cross-sectional research on the factors that influence how families' function indicates mixed results. These factors are the severity of the child's disability and family characteristics, health, support, and family hardiness. Several studies suggest that families with psychological problems score lower on family functioning than control groups (Baigas, 2002; Friedmann et al., 1997; Keitner et al., 1991; Keitner, Miller, & Ryan, 1993; Miller, Epstein, Bishop, & Keitner, 1985). Other studies have not supported these findings (Epstein et al., 1993; Kim, 2002) and there has been little information about cultural influences on family functioning (Roncone et al., 1998; Shek, 2002; Stevenson-Hinde & Akister, 1995). Therefore, research is needed to better understand how Taiwanese DMD families function.

Purpose of the Study

The overall purpose of this study was to explore the factors associated with functioning among Taiwanese families with a child having DMD. The specific aims to achieve the purposes of this study were as follows:

1. Describe the child's level of disability, access to care, and family characteristics.

2. Describe family health, family hardiness, family support, and family functioning experienced by the parents with DMD children.

3. Describe the relationship among DMD child's level of disability and access to care (age when diagnosed with DMD), family health, family characteristics (family employment and family annual income), family supports, family hardiness, and family functioning.

4. Determine how the child's level of disability and access to care, family health, family characteristics, family support, and family hardiness predicted family functioning in families with a DMD child

5. Test the model of Family Stressors, Resources, and Functioning with families with a child with DMD.

Summary

Little is understood about how families function when they have a child with DMD. Several studies focused on the impact and coping of families with disabled children. Given the research gaps, and lack of information about the functioning of culturally diverse families with a disabled child, this study involved a group of Taiwanese families to discover whether the factors associated with family functioning found in the literature were characteristic of them.

Family Functioning and the Resiliency Model

Definition of Family

The family is a complex system of interacting individuals who share a history and a future. Families consist of structures, roles, and functions (McGoldrick & Carter, 2003). Family structure is the number of members of the family; family roles include parents, spouse, child, other kin, etc.; and family functions involve the ability to satisfy members' physical, psychological, survival, and maintenance needs (Smith, 1995).

Definition of Family Functioning

The basic attributes of family functioning are characterized and explained by how a family system typically appraises, operates, and behaves (McCubbin & Thompson, 1991). Family functioning also includes the ability to solve problems. The ability to maintain a balance between change and stability is another aspect of healthy family functioning (Olson, 1993).

Family functioning is a reliable predictor of parental adjustment and adaptation. Normal functioning refers to the ability to achieve family goals, meet situational and developmental challenges, and adjust to economic circumstances and cultural norms (Walsh, 1993). The important attributes of healthy family functioning include commitment, responsibility, organizational stability, adaptability, communication, problem solving, belief system, and resources (Walsh, 1993). Healthy family functioning does not mean absence of problems, but rather "the healthy family can be found in the midst problems as in family resilience" (Walsh, 2003, p. 5). Therefore, the presence of distress is not necessarily a criterion of family pathology (Epstein et al., 1993).

Definition of Family Resilience

Resilience is the ability to function well and to be competent when faced with life stress. Resiliency is "the family's ability to use their existing strengths and resources to overcome crises and to react positively to challenges" (Berry, 2004, para 3). McCubbin, Thompson, and McCubbin (2001) defined resiliency as:

> the positive behavioral patterns and functional competence individuals and the family unit demonstrate under stressful or adverse circumstances, which determine the family's ability to recover by maintaining its integrity as a unit, the well being of family members and the family unit. (p. 5)

It is encouraging to note that some families' ability to adapt to stress leads to higher than normal levels of functioning (Patterson, 2002). McCubbin and McCubbin (1988) defined family resilience as "characteristics, dimensions, and properties of families which help families to be resistant to disruption in the face of crisis situations" (p. 247). The institute for Health and Disability (1997) states that

> A "resilient family" can balance the demands of the child with a chronic condition with other family needs, maintain clear family boundaries, develop communication competence, attribute positive meanings to the situation, maintain family flexibility, maintain a commitment to the family, engage in active coping efforts, maintain social integration, and develop collaborative relationships with professionals. (p. 6)

Resiliency Model of Family Stress, Adjustment, and Adaptation

The Resiliency Model of Family Stress, Adjustment, and Adaptation (figure 1), which is derived from a substantial body of research (McCubbin et al., 2001; McCubbin & McCubbin, 1993) on family functioning over time, emerges from studies of war-induced family crises, the study of families faced with chronic stressors and illness (Kosciulek, McCubbin, & McCubbin, 1993) and the study of native Hawaiian, Filipino, Asian, American, and African-American families faced with both normative and nonnormative stressors and crises (McCubbin et al., 2001). Therefore, the Resiliency Model may be helpful to understand the ability to function among families who have a child with DMD.

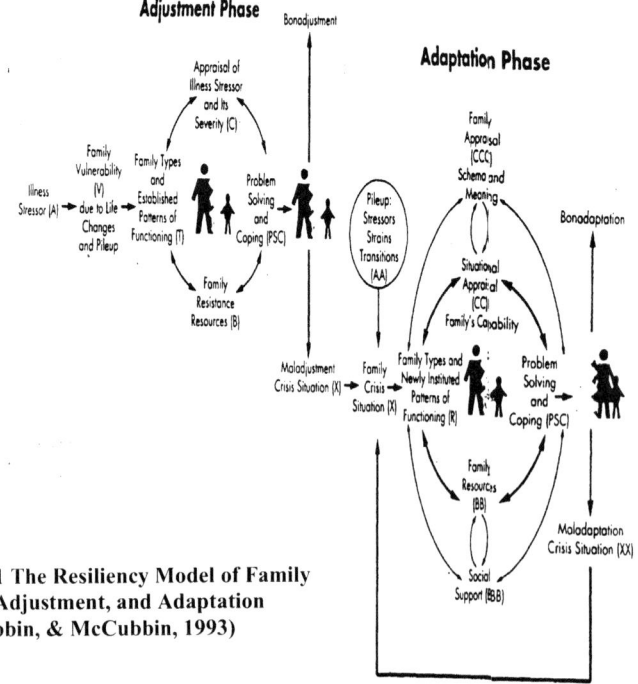

Figure 1 The Resiliency Model of Family Stress, Adjustment, and Adaptation (McCubbin, & McCubbin, 1993)

The resiliency model is characterized as having two discernible phases: adjustment and adaptation (McCubbin, McCubbin, Thompson, & Thompson, 1998). The traits of family adjustment and adaptation are healthy, normal, invulnerable, and resilient in well-functioning families. The Resiliency Model (McCubbin & McCubbin, 1993) characterizes the family system as "a resources exchange network in which problem solving and coping are the actions for this exchange" (p. 55). Successful family adaptation is achieved when "family schema and patterns of functioning are congruent, family members' personality and growth are supported, the family 's relationship with the community is mutually supportive, and the family develops a shared sense of coherence" (p. 59). Family adaptation involves the process of restructuring and making changes in rules, boundaries, and patterns of functioning. Families who experience an excessive demand from stressors deplete their resources; but when they adapt, they can restore functional stability and promote family satisfaction (McCubbin et al., 2001).

Families of children with DMD who are resilient may able to adjust to changing circumstances and have a positive attitude toward the challenges of family life. Bonadjustment (successful adjustments) occur when the needs of individual family members are met, and functioning of the family system and its transaction with the community is not threatened. However, having a child with DMD places enormous burdens upon how families function. The disability experience affects the functioning of the whole family, creating intense stress and draining its total resources. The chronic stress may result in disruption and break down of the family's functioning when the demands on the physical and psychological energy and other resources are too great. This outcome is termed maladjustment.

Family capabilities may be inadequate to deal with the chronic hardships of DMD leading to maladjustment and crisis (McCubbin et al., 2001). A family in crisis may try to develop new patterns of functioning, marking the beginning of the second phase of the Resiliency Model, the adaptation phase (McCubbin et al., 2001). During the adaptation phase, associated stressors as severe as the disability of the DMD child may produce a pile-up of demands with the family becoming increasing vulnerable. At this point, the family engages in dynamic relational processes to introduce changes in existing patterns of functioning to help resolve stressors. The family's level of appraisal influences the family system, and affects patterns of functioning, problem solving, and coping (McCubbin et al., 2001). A family that adapts to stress in these ways leads to a higher level of functioning.

Family adaptation is the optimal outcome if a new level of balance, harmony, coherence, and a satisfactory level of functioning is achieved following the progression of a disability (McCubbin et al., 2001). The adaptation phase of the Resiliency Model differs from the adjustment phase in that the family must develop new patterns of functioning in order to successfully adapt to their situation; if not, the Resiliency Model suggests that there will be a deterioration of the family's integrity, autonomy, or ability to manage their current crisis (McCubbin et al., 2001). There are several components of this model that can determine whether families can adapt. Each of these components is discussed below.

Family Stressors

Stressors may threaten the stability of the family unit or place significant demands on the family's resources and capabilities (McCubbin et al., 2001). McCubbin et al. (2001) used the Family Inventory of Life Events and Changes to measure family stressors and strains.

Family Resources

Family resources are a family's capabilities and strengths to resist a crisis and achieve harmony and balance. Hardiness is another term that represents these capabilities and strengths. Hardiness is a manifestation of competence despite exposure to significant stressors, and is another measure of healthy family functioning. Hardiness is a term that was first identified as personal resilience (eg. health status), characterized by commitment, challenge, and control (Kobasa, 1979). Hardiness results from "resilience processes that contribute to family dynamics and the family's abilities to cope effectively and adapt in crises" (Cohen, Slonim, Finzi, & Leichtentritt, 2002, p. 183). The components of family resilience include interpersonal relationships, open emotional sharing, system flexibility to shift roles and provide support, connectedness, and family values. McCubbin et al. (2001) refer "family hardiness" to

> The internal strengths and durability of the family unit and is characterized
> by a sense of control over the outcomes of life events and hardships, a
> view of change as beneficial and growth producing, and an active rather
> than passive orientation in adjusting to and managing stressful situations.
> (p. 274)

Hardy families "shared a commitment to each other", "coped with change", "cultivated a protective environment in which family members actively" promoted "esteem among each other and themselves", "developed healthy lifestyles", and "encouraged coping skills of individual members" (Thames & Thomason, 2000, p. 1)

The Family Hardiness Index, the Family Inventory of Resources for Management, and the Family Time and Routines Index have often been used to measure the characteristics of hardiness as a stress resistor and adaptation resource that reflects the internal strengths and durability of the family unit (McCubbin et al., 2001).

Family Problem Solving and Coping

Family problem solving and coping indicate actions that reflect a family's ability to deal with stressors and hardship to maintain or restore family harmony and balance. Researchers often use the Coping Health Inventory for Parents (CHIP), the Family Crisis Oriented Personal Evaluation Scales (F-COPES), and the Family Problem Solving Communication scale (FPSC) to measure the extent of family coping ability (McCubbin, McCubbin, & Thompson, 1996).

Family Appraisal

Family appraisal is the family's perception of the seriousness of a stressor and its effects. It addresses family beliefs and expectations regarding the stressor and is defined as a familial sense of coherence. Appraisal has been measured using the Family Sense of Coherence (Antonovsky & Sourani, 1988).

Family Schema and Meaning

Family schema is "a structure of fundamental convictions, values, beliefs, and expectations" (McCubbin, Thompson, Thompson, Elver, & McCubbin, 1998, p. 42). A family schema includes cultural-ethical beliefs and values. Family schema is how families attach meanings to their situation. The meaning is often determined by spiritual values and beliefs. Family schema assists the development of meaning through the processes of affirmation and spiritualization. Family schema have been measured using the Family (Ethnicity) Schema Index (McCubbin et al., 2001; McCubbin, Thompson et al., 1998).

Family Adaptation

Family adaptation is the outcome of the family's efforts to create new ways of functioning in response to family stressors and is characterized as the minimal discrepancy between demands and capabilities (McCubbin et al., 2001). Family adaptation results "in a new or satisfactory level of balance, harmony, and functioning to a crisis situation" (McCubbin et al., 2001, p. 74). Family adaptation is often measured using the Family Assessment Device.

Research on Family Resilience

A review of studies on family resilience identifies four factors that influence family adaptation and three groups of factors that affect family functioning in families with a disabled child. Factors influencing adaptation include (a) stress related to emotional climate and pessimism concerning the child's future, (b) sense of coherence and use of resources, (c) social support, and (d) family strengths. Family hardiness, family support, and family communication; family problem solving communication, family schema, and family meaning; and family time together, life style, and accumulation of stressors and strains influence family functioning.

Factors Influencing Family Adaptation

Stress related to emotional climate and pessimism concerning the child's future. Dyson (1997) found that there was no difference between fathers and mothers of children with disabilities in levels of parental stress, social support, or family functioning. Parental stress was related to family problems resulting from the child's special needs, the family's emotional climate, and parents' pessimism concerning the child's future. The high rate of parent-reported child behavior problems among children with disabilities could reflect parental distress, especially about impairment in the social skills of their children (Smith & Oliver, 2001). Nereo et al. (2003) found that disabled children's emotional behavior problems were associated with mothers' stress. Psychosocial stressors in the lives of the mothers of children with handicapping conditions may result in initial shock, crisis, emotional changes, and pressures on family and social roles, requiring adjustment of parental role expectations (Burden, 1991).

Sabbeth (1984) found that fathers were at special risk for developing feelings of helplessness in relation to a child with a disability because of a number of conditions. Seligman and Daring (1989) also indicated that fathers and mothers also differ in their initial response to the diagnosis of a child who is disabled. In addition, Damrosch and Perry (1989) noted that fathers and mothers differed with regard to adjustment patterns and coping behaviors, and Ptacek, Smith, and Zanas (1992) found that men and women cope differently with stress.

Sense of coherence and use of resources. Bristor (1991) noted that quality of life for physically disabled children may depend to a large degree on the parents' ability to care for the child completely. In addition, socio-economic or material resources, locus of control, self-esteem, relationships with the family and social network, and service response can improve adaptation (Knussen & Sloper, 1992).

Gottlieb's (1998) research emphasized stress and coping resources in single- mothers of school-age children with a variety of developmental disabilities. In a study of 152 single mothers with developmentally disabled children, he found that their sense of coherence (life as comprehensible, manageable, and meaningful) was associated with family adaptation. Single mothers who had a strong sense of coherence and greater use of resources had more adaptive outcomes. The sense of coherence was related to the mothers' perceptions of their child with disabilities.

Lustig (1997) studied 116 parents of adult children with mental retardation and found that most were resilient and exhibited positive functioning. There were positive correlations between scores on family adaptation and social support, family sense of coherence, and family adaptability. Lustig's work led to an empirical family typology and knowledge of a family's sense of coherence.

Margalit and Yona (1991) compared the ability of family systems to cope (including perception of family climate and sense of coherence) in an Israeli kibbutz (49 families with nondisabled children and 43 families with disabled children) and in an Israeli city (48 families of disabled children, 51 families of non-disabled children). The findings indicated that parents' sense of coherence assisted them to develop effective parental skills for seeking solutions to their child's specific needs. The implication was that improving parents' perception of coherence would promote family strength.

Social support. Judge (1998) examined the relationship between parental perceptions of coping strategies and family strength in 69 parents of young Caucasian children with disabilities in one geographic region. The results showed that use of social support was highly associated with family strength. This study provides evidence that families' informal and formal sources of support can strengthen family adaptation.

Bennett and Deluca (1996) used in-depth interviews of 12 parents with a disabled child to investigate the use of networks. Results showed that parents got (a) emotional support and caregiving from families and friends; (b) emotional outlets and sources of information from parent groups; and (c) ideas for action and support from professionals. The implication is that a social network has an effect on family adaptation.

McCubbin, McCubbin, and Thompson (1993) conducted a study of the impact of pressures, strengths, and capacities on family life with 200 families in Hawaii including Caucasian (N=78), Asian (N=49), Hawaiian (N=37), and mixed-race families (N=36). The results showed that social support appeared to have greater explanatory power than other indexes for family adaptation. The major strength of the study is that it used a random digit dialing process and the sample size was large enough to compare the impact of disability on families in four different races. A second strength is that the study identified the reliability and validity of each psychometric measure of family adaptation. The third strength is that the findings of the study supported two critical explanatory factors, family schema and appraisal in the Resiliency Model.

Family strengths. McIntyre (2000) examined the role of competency-enhancing help in the adaptation process for 77 mothers of children with special needs. They found that higher levels of competency-enhancing help were related to greater maternal adaptation as measured by maternal sense of well-being and satisfaction with family functioning. In addition, competency-enhancing help was positively related to family resources and the use of positive coping strategies.

Silberberg (2001) used multiple methods to study 605 families and found that self-identified strong families agreed with positive statements (e.g., strongly connected to each other, easily to share values and ideas, love one another, often laugh with each other, enjoy helping each other) (p. 53). She found eight qualities of family strength among 177 volunteers including communication, togetherness, commitment, sharing activities, affection, support, acceptance, and resilience. She also extracted two strong themes from 33 families: support from extended family and friends and positive co-parenting arrangements. The major implication for nursing is a strengths-based approach that focuses on available resources and skills within the family and community, and the empowerment of the family and community in building resilience.

Factors Influencing Family Functioning

Family hardiness, family support, and family communication. Olsen, et al. (1999) studied 54 couples (108 parents) of young children with disabilities and found that income, family support, and incendiary communication (defined as communication that is inflammatory in nature and tends to exacerbate stressful situations) predicted parent's hardiness. McCubbin, McCubbin and Thompson (1996) found that family hardiness was positively related to family support for the mothers and fathers, but negatively related to incendiary communication. Based on their findings, the researchers suggest that families develop basic capabilities and strengths, which foster the development and growth of family members and protect them from major disruption during family changes or transitions.

Family problem solving communication, family schema, and family meaning. McCubbin, Thompson et al. (1998) gathered self-report data from 101 parents of Native Hawaiian preschool children. Results showed that poor family problem solving, communication, and lack of family hardiness to be significant predictors of family dysfunction. Family schema was indirectly related to family dysfunction, primarily through coherence, hardiness, and family problem-solving communication. The authors constructed a series of path models to account for indirect relationships of family schema and sense of coherence on levels of family functioning. A major strength of this study was the use of the Resiliency Model as the basis of the study and use of a randomly selected sample, thus making it a more reliable representation of the intended population of Native Hawaiians. But the small sample size limits generalizability of the findings.

Cannors' and Donnella's (1998) anthropological study explored parents' perceptions and coping abilities in eight Navajo families with autistic children and 24 families without autism. Results showed that parents were concerned about their children's social competency and residential placement. The implications are that professionals should encourage the family to become involved in early childhood special education, advocate for a family-centered approach, look at their own expectations, provide a loving and caring relationship, to protect the child.

Garwick, Kohrman, Titus, Wolman, and Blum (1999) designed a grounded theory study of 63 family caregivers of school children with chronic physical health impairments and used the Impact-on-Family Scale to discover how Hispanic, African-American, and European American families explain the cause of childhood chronic conditions and the indicators of resilience reflected in these explanations. The categories of explanation for the cause of childhood chronic conditions were: biomedical and environmental explanations, traditional and fatalistic beliefs, cause unknown, and personal attributions.

The major strength of the study is that the impact of traditional ethnocultural beliefs on families' explanations is most evident in descriptions of folk beliefs about illness and religious/spiritual interpretations of the chronic conditions. The influence of culture is also apparent in expressions of fatalistic and superstitious beliefs that reflect the family's worldview, thus contributing the development of a substantive theory. A second strength is related to the development and refinement of psychometric measures focused on the impact of attitudes and ethnic differences. The third major strength is the contribution to our understanding of family explanations of their knowledge and attitudes toward minority patients and on the families' perceptions of cross-cultural health care behaviors. An important contribution of this research is a greater awareness and sensitivity of cultural differences in the meaning the family attributes to the cause of the child's condition.

Cohen et al. (2002) used a qualitative grounded theory method to study fifteen Israeli women whose families underwent crisis events. The authors found that family abilities, flexibility to shift roles, and the willingness of family members to give up their personal needs for someone else and to accept other people's feelings promoted family resilience. Other contributing factors included a sense of humor, trust, and providing a sense of security. The implications from this study focused on improving communication. However, the sample size was small and did not include males so the ability to generalize findings is limited.

Family time together, life style, pile-up of stressors and strains. McCubbin (1998) used regression analysis with data gathered from 184 African American enlisted military personnel and their spouses to determine factors most influential in helping them adjust to overseas assignments. Military life style (coherence) and confidence in spouse's self-reliance, spouse employment, and spouse's assessment of family time together emerged as important factors associated with family functioning. Critical variables of the accumulation of stressors and strains, and particularly family strengths, support, and coherence were of central importance in explaining African-American enlisted family functioning in the face of reassignment.

Finally, Hawley (2000) based his study on the family resilience and narrative therapy model. Barriers to effective family communication and relationships were finances, differences over religion, father's depression, and interference from mother's ex-husband. A focus on family strengths and successes, developmental path, overcoming obstacles to achieve well - being, and obtaining outside resources led to improved family functioning.

These studies represent a wide variety of disciplines including epidemiology, sociology, psychology, and psychiatry. Most studies identified a broad range of background conditions, personal characteristics, social relations and community resources that may be helpful to understanding family functioning among DMD families. Many of these studies support various aspects of the Resiliency Model. In addition, the studies often explored the concept of resilience from multiple family dimensional processes including belief systems, organizational patterns, and communication processes. Family functioning research has contributed to a recognition of the need for interventions, such as personal or social support networks, self-help groups based on conventional wisdom, strength-based approaches to family support to facilitate family functioning. However, the Resiliency Model cannot be used to measure the family adaptation of Taiwanese families because there are no reliability and validity measures in Mandarin to assess the several aspects of the model (e.g. family appraisal, schema, and meaning). Furthermore, the model does not consider the inherited, progressive, life-threatening nature of a condition like DMD as a family stressor. Therefore, a modified version of the model was used to examine the family functioning of DMD families in this study.

Conceptual Model of Family Stressors, Resources, and Functioning

The Conceptual Model of Family Stressors, Resources, and Functioning is proposed in Figure 2 and includes the measured concepts (variables), and empirical indicators (instruments). Figure 2, represents the relationship among the variables of family stressors, resources, and functioning. Independent variables were the child's disability and access to care. The dependent variable was family functioning. The mediating variables were family health, family characteristics, family support, and family hardiness. Family health, family characteristics, family support, and family hardiness are consequences of a child's disability and antecedents of family function.

A brief discussion of each variable and its relationship to the other variables will be presented next.

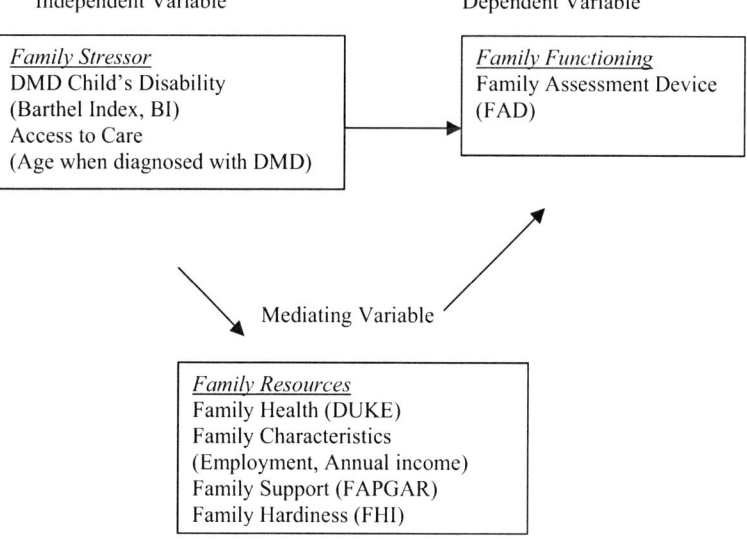

Figure 2 Conceptual Models for Family Stressors, Resources, and Functioning

Family Stressors

In the Model, family stressors (the child's disability and access to care) place demands on family resources. As the DMD child's condition worsens the families may become more vulnerable. Families in crisis try to resolve stressors by using family resources, reviewing the meaning of life, and engaging in dynamic relational processes to guide changes in existing patterns of family functioning to resolve their stressors (McCubbin & McCubbin, 1993). The following literature review will focus on terminology, measurement and their relationship to family functioning.

Child's disability. Disability means an incapacity or disqualification. A child with a disability is deprived of physical or mental abilities. It is a long-term impairment adversely affecting specific normal daily activities (Kenneth, 2001). A disability makes the DMD children depend on families to give them assistance and that stressors contributes to an accumulation of demands on the families. Holroyd and Guthrie (1979) reported that physical incapacitation of chronically ill children with neuromuscular or psychiatric disease was a predictor of burden. Snowdon, Cameron, and Dunham (1994) found that severity of child's condition and behavior problems are the significant stressors for the families with developmental disabilities. The severity of disability was defined on the child's independence, measured by the Barthel Index, to evaluate daily activity conditions.

The Barthel Index (BI) is probably the most widely used generic disability measure. It was developed in 1955 as a simple index of independence useful in scoring disability. Independence means that the person needs no assistance at any part of the task (Mahoney & Barthel, 1965). The BI was as good as any other single simple index for clinical purposes but might be limited in the context of research (Wade & Collin, 1988). Van der Putten, Hobart, Freeman, and Thompson (1999) suggested that the Functional Independence Measure had no advantages over the BI in evaluating changes in disability due to therapeutic interventions. This has important clinical implications, as the BI is quicker and simpler to rate.

Access to care. Once children are diagnosed with DMD, their parents are in continual contact with health professionals regardless of the children's age. Generally, the parents will gather or research formal knowledge about the disease from professional and begin to access supportive care system when children are diagnosed. Care assists the process of emotional adjustment to the child's disability, enabling parents to access service and benefits, and improve parents' management of the child's behavior (Pain, 1999). Only after diagnosis do parents learn what information is helpful (Pain, 1999). Some parents felt that information was hard to get because they didn't know the right question to ask (Beresford, 1994). Some researchers have concluded that professionals can provide support to parents by providing resources and expertise and helping create and maintain an open, honest, and collaborative relationship with parents (Bennett & DeLuca, 1996; McCallion & Toseland, 1993). This study identified the age when a child was diagnosed with DMD, noting that earlier detection implied families had early access to professional care.

Family Resources

Family resources are the capacities of families to respond to the crisis of their child's illness so they can regenerate personal energy (McCubbin et al., 2001). Snowdon et al. (1994) suggest that hardiness, health, esteem, and communication are coping resources. The components of family resources in the proposed Model include family characteristics (employment and family annual income), family health, family support, and family hardiness. These are viewed as mediating variables that provide family energy to address each member's physical, mental, social, and spiritual needs in order to solve problems and maintain healthy family functioning.

Family health. To bring an ill, handicapped, or disabled child into the world is one of the most heartbreaking events parents ever face. Chronic emotional stress was reported by parents to be the most significant problem in coping with a child who has DMD due to the unrelenting, constant demands of medical, physical and emotional care required by the disease. There is no doubt that the physical, psychological, social, and emotional health and well-being of family members are essential protective and recovery factors in promoting resilience in families (McCubbin, McCubbin, Thompson, Han, & Allen, 1997) and are often used as the outcome measure of resiliency (McCubbin et al., 1997). Therefore, the degree of family health may explain the variability in resiliency in the family system. Parkerson, Broadhead, and Tse (1991) developed the Duke Health Profile (Duke) to measure self-reported health, quality of life, and functional health status. It has been used primarily for research on health-related outcomes in the clinical setting. In this study family health parental health, measured by the Duke Health Profile, to evaluate physical, social, mental, perceived health, anxiety, depression, disability, self-esteem, and pain.

Family characteristics. Family characteristics are a family's capabilities and strengths to resist a crisis and promote family resilience to maintain patterns of functioning to achieve harmony and balance. Based on Smilkstein's (1978) acronym SCREEM-the major family characteristics are social, culture, religious, economic, educational and medical. When families have social support, cultural satisfaction, economic stability, high education, and access to medical care, they are better able to function.

As DMD progresses, demands upon the parents also increase. The financial burden of a chronically ill child falls most heavily on middle-class Taiwanese families because parents are often searching for alternative therapy that is not covered by insurance. Palfrey et al. (1989) found that educational level and socioeconomic factors had significant effects on parental stress. Reid and Renwick (2001) found that familial stress is not significantly related to any of the socio-demographic measures. But Canning, Harris, and Kelleher (1996) reported that family stress was related to family income. Svavarsdottir (1997) found that the number of children and family income were positively correlated with family hardiness, indicating mothers of children with asthma who had more children and higher income reported higher hardiness (r = .27). There was no relationship between family hardiness and parents' age, and length of marriage. So, parents' employment and annual income were the most important variables of family characteristics in the model.

Family support. Family support is family members' satisfaction with their family's responsiveness and caring for their needs. These include adaptation, partnership, growth, affection, and resolve. Family support services can encourage the use of cognitive coping strategies to facilitate healthy functioning in families with disabled children (Summers, Behr, & Turnbull, 1989). Yu (2002) used the Family APGAR (FAPGAR) to evaluate family support and found that there was a positive correlation with self-efficacy for the families of tuberculosis patients. Some researchers translated the FAPGAR into Mandarin as"家庭關懷度指數 chia ting guan huai du zhi shu" that retranslated into English means "family caring index" (Smilkstein, 1978). A low score was shown to be predictive of psychosocial problems in children, patients, and families (Chen, 1988; Chen, Chen, Hsu, & Lin, 1980; Tsai, Chang, & Tseng, 1993; Tyan, Chie, & Chang, 1988). This study used the meaning of "family caring index" to measure perceived family support in the five domains of adaptation, partnership, growth, affection, and resolve (Gardner et al., 2001).

Family hardiness. Family hardiness is the internal strength of a family system and durability of family unit characterized by a sense of control to over life events and hardships by the family working together to solve problems. Leske (2003) defined "hardiness as the family's internal strengths and durability" that help a family adapt over time by "an ability to work together to find solutions to difficulties" (p. 33). Lambert and Lambert (1999) defined "hardiness as a constellation of attitudes, beliefs, and behavioral tendencies that consist of three components: commitment, control, and challenge" (p. 11).

For this study, family hardiness was conceptualized as the energy resource used to help facilitate adjustment and adaptation over time by serving to release the negative effects of stressors and demands. In addition, being able to view change as beneficial and growth-producing and an active rather than passive orientation in adjusting to and managing stressful situations is also important to family hardiness. The attributes of family hardiness include commitment, challenge, and control (McCubbin et al., 2001). Family hardiness is a mediating factor to decrease the effects of stressors and demands on the family and maintain normal family functioning.

McCubbin, et al. (2001) developed "the Family Hardiness Index (FHI) to measure the characteristics of hardiness as a stress resistance resource and adaptation resource in families, which would function as a buffer or mediating factor of stressors and demands and as a facilitation of family adjustment and adaptation" (p. 274). Henkle (1994) found that family hardiness is an important resistant resource for the burden and stress of family caregiving. Kamya (1997) found that family hardiness would explain the variance in caregiver well-being and suggested that future research should be on caregivers of the functionally impaired. Donnelly (1994) reported that parents of children with asthma viewed their families as hardy, and found that there was a significant relationship between family hardiness and family coherence and adaptability, but no relationship between family hardiness and family stress.

Olsen, et al. (1999) used hardiness to describe people who remained healthy even while experiencing high amounts of life stress. They defined hardiness as the sum of 3 components: control, commitment, and challenge, just as Lambert and Lambert (1999) did. A few studies have explored the construct of family hardiness (Failla & Jones, 1991; McCubbin, Thompson, & McCubbin, 1996) and influencing factors that included family stress, family support, emotional distress, family coping strategies, family appraisal, and demographic factors (Campbell & Demi, 2000; Mellon & Northouse, 2001; Olsen et al., 1999).

Mellon and Northouse (2001) explored the quality of life of families of long-term survivors of a cancer; they found that there was significant positive relationship between family hardiness and family quality of life ($r = .37$); significant negative relationships between family hardiness and family stressors ($r = -.26$); and family hardiness and patients' fear of recurrence ($r = -.24$). Family hardiness made a unique contribution to the variance in family meaning of the cancer illness.

Family Functioning

Family functioning is the outcome of the families' ability to use family resources and other sources of support. In this study, problem solving, communication, role, affective responsiveness, affective involvement, behavior control, and healthy family functioning were conceptualized as attributes of the resilient DMD family (Epstein, Bishop, Ryan, Miller, & Keitner, 2003). In addition, family health, family support and family hardiness were viewed as indicators of adaptation of the DMD family. Successful family functioning has been found to reduce demands on the family system and brings resources to manage the situation (McCubbin et al., 2001).

Several different attributes of family functioning have been described. Epstein, Bishop, and Levin (1978) defined them as problem solving, communication, role, affective responsiveness, affective involvement, and behavior control. Olson, Sprenkle, and Russell (1979) identified the attributes of family functioning as family cohesion, adaptability, and communication; Beavers and Hampson (1993) described them as competence and style; Suttiamnuaykul (2001) noted that basic attributes appropriate to culture, society, economic, and political policy were important for families to function well.

Family functioning has been studied among families with children with various serious conditions, resulting in conflicting findings. For example, some studies report a negative relationship between family functioning and the children's conditions: major depressive disorders, depression (Fornari, Wlodarczyk-Bisaga, Matthews, Sandberg, & Katz, 1999; Stein et al., 2000; Tamplin & Goodyer, 2001), suicide adolescent depression (King, Segal, Naylor, & Evans, 1993), psychiatric disorders (Friedmann et al., 1997), eating disorders of bulima nervosa (Fornari et al., 1999), anorexia nervosa (Gowers & North, 1999), mental retardation, down syndrome, physical disability (Luescher, Dede, Gitten, Fennell, & Maria, 1999), epilepsy (Pal, Chaudhury, Das, & Sengupta, 2002), traumatic brain injury (Rivara et al., 1996), or oppositional defiant disorder (Tamplin, Goodyer, & Herbert, 1998). Other studies found that there were no relationships between the children's condition and family functioning: fractures (Loder, Warschausky, Schwartz, Hensinger, & Greenfield, 1995), developmental disability (Dyson, 1997), or anorexia nervosa (Dare & Key, 1999) - in family functioning. There were no significant differences between parents from families with healthy and unhealthy children (Keitner et al., 1995). Furthermore, the severity of involvement of cerebral palsy children did not seem to influence parents' perception of family functioning (Magill-Evans, Darrah, Pain, Adkins, & Kratochvil, 2001).

Early studies of family functioning focused on the family's economic functioning. The pioneer LePlay (Silver, 1982), who conducted the first study of family functioning in the 1850s, submitted that family functioning was related to health and well-being of the family. His research was based on analysis of family budgets. Other pioneer studies of family functioning supported LePlay's important idea of economic functioning (Schwab, Gray-Ice, & Prentice, 2000). After 1859, some family research focused on hereditary influences on mental health and illness that were related to procreative and social functioning of the family. These studies pointed to the importance of the family's basic reproductive function.

At the end of the 20th century, abortion, family values, and day care became the key issues and replaced reproductive functioning. Researchers were interested in hereditary patterns of mental illness and mental retardation in the family. Families of patients with depression were likely to experience more dysfunction than families without psychiatric disorders (Friedmann et al., 1997; Keitner et al., 1991; Keitner et al., 1993). Fifty to seventy percent of families of depressed patients perceived their own family functioning as unhealthy (Keitner et al., 1995).

Lately, repeated studies have found the negative effects of depression or chronic mental illness on family well-being. Keitner (1990) found significant associations between depressed patients and the quality of family functioning, especially impaired role functioning. Friedmann et al., (1997) found that "having a family member in an acute phase of psychiatric illness was a risk factor for poor family functioning" (p.357). And 80% of the families with anxiety disorders and 74.8% of the families with major depression had unhealthy functioning in communication, with 50-80% of the various patients' families with impaired general function.

The correlation between behavioral–emotional symptoms and family dysfunction has been found in other studies (Heru & Ryan, 2002; Keitner, Ryan, Miller, & Norman, 1992; Lindeman et al., 2002). Scahill et al. (1999) found that children with attention-deficit hyperactivity disorder (ADHD) were more likely to live in low-income families with higher levels of family dysfunction. Poor family functioning at 5 years after a child was sexually abused was associated with low self-esteem and behavior problems (Tebbutt, Swanston, Oates, & O'Toole, 1997).

Acreman (2002) found that gender of child, family income, single parent status, parental level of education, family functioning, parental depression and school readiness as predictors of academic resilience. Baigas (2002) indicated that lower rates of visual-motor,

academic, adaptive, and social development after four months were found in children whose
families scored more dysfunctional on the FAD. And there were significant differences
between learning disability (LD) and non-LD families on structure and interaction on five of
the seven FAD scales: roles, behavior control, communication, affective-responsiveness, and
general functioning. However, there was a positive relationship between healthy family
functioning and socioeconomic level. Vandsburger (2001) suggested that the effects of
family hardiness and social support on family functioning in families experiencing economic
pressure did not fit these data.

Kim (2002) found that intra-family and extra-family resources were significant
predictors of family functioning. Whether the child had a disability and the age of the child
(adolescent versus young adult) were not significant predictors. Researchers have found that
dyadic relationships within the family, especially parent-child relationship, are related to the
functioning of the family (Hayden et al., 1998).

Conclusion

The disability of the DMD child induces the family to change and experience many
challenges over their life-time, putting their family functioning at-risk. A complete
understanding of how well DMD families' function, however, is unknown. With little
information about Taiwanese family functioning in general, and conflicting data about the
functioning of families with seriously ill children from in larger populations, further research
is needed.

The DMD population in Taiwan has been studied to improve understanding of family
stress, parents' coping, social support, and quality of life (Chen et al., 2002; Chen et al., 2003;
Huang & Dai, 1998; Kao, 1998). However, knowledge about family support, family
hardiness, and family functioning in the DMD family is needed before health care
professionals can provide family-centered interventions that promote family health,
adaptation, and better family functioning.

METHODOLOGY

This descriptive correlational study used a cross-sectional, predictive design to explore the family functioning of 126 parents aged 28 to 61 years in Taiwan who have a child with DMD. The design looked at an event at one specific point in time (Rubin & Babbie, 1997). The study used the Conceptual Model of Stressors, Resources, and Functioning (Figure 2), a revised version of the Resiliency Model, because several instruments used for the latter have not been tested or translated into Mandarin. For example, only one subscale of the Family Hardiness Index, has been translated.

Table 1 showed the concepts, variables, and instruments in the present study. Child's disability and access to care were measured by self-report. The degree of the child's disability and reported age when diagnosed with DMD were the family stressors. Family resources included family characteristics, family health status, family support, and family hardiness. These were measured with a demographic sheet including parents' employment and family annual income, the scales of the individual Duke Health Profile (Duke), the Family APGAR (FAPGAR), and the Family Hardiness Index (FHI). Family functioning was measured with a scale of the individual Family Assessment Device (FAD). All instruments were translated into the Chinese language and used in Taiwan. This study utilized the data collected from the parents. Participants individually completed each measurement. They were excluded if the DMD children, siblings, or grandparents helped parents answer the questionnaires.

Table 1

Concepts, Variables, and Instruments in the Current Study

Concepts	Variables	Instruments
Family Stressors	Child Disability	
	Daily activity dependent	Barthel Index (BI)
	Access to Care	Demographic Sheet
	Age when diagnosed	
	with DMD	
Family Resources	Family Health	Duke health profile (DUKE)
	Family Hardiness	Family Hardiness Index (FHI)
	Family Support	Family APGAR (FAPGAR)
	Family Characteristics	Demographic Sheet
	Family annual income	
	Parents' employment	
Family Functioning	Family Functioning	Family Assessment Device (FAD)

Identification of Study Population

The study used a convenience sample to recruit parents of children with DMD into the study. Although convenience samples have advantages for multiple reasons including recruiting time, accessibility, and low expense, there was a chance that respondents might not have returned the questionnaires if they hadn't received a follow-up phone call, a stamped return envelope, and assurance of confidential communication. In addition, the sample may not have been representative of the population and those who were more uncomfortable might have refused to participate in the study. The question of generalizability was addressed (Polit & Hunger, 1999), in part, by having a representative sample of parents from each of the families with DMD children in the Taiwan Muscular Dystrophy Association (TMDA). Therefore, results can be generalized only to the DMD group of the TMDA (86.4% of the participants were members of this organization).

The target population for this study were parents of children with DMD who participated in TMDA's groups or used medical resources from Kaohsiung Medical University Hospital (KMU hospital) for diagnostic evaluation, support, and medical care. Pediatric neurologists diagnosed the children's DMD through muscle biopsy and serological tests (creatine phosphokinase-CPK and lactate dehydrogenase-LDH) and provided follow-up care. The TMDA, created in 1995, developed support groups for DMD families and expanded to other families with family members with different types of muscle dystrophy. There were three branches of the organization, located in the south, north, and central areas of Taiwan.

Subject Sample

A convenience sample of 126 parents participated in this study. They came from a total pool of 125 DMD families (245 parents) in the TMDA, as well as outpatients from Kaohsiung Medical University (KMU) hospital. The response rate to questionnaires was 62% (based on mailings to 203 parents who had agreed to receive the questionnaires). Forty-six couples (58%) completed the questionnaires; eight fathers (10% of families), and 26 mothers (32% of families) also completed the questionnaires. The subjects who declined to participate had multiple reasons, including death, divorce, separation, illness; others had no forwarding address or gave no reason.

Demographic Description of the Subjects

The demographic characteristics of the 126 parents are found in Table 2. The majority of parents were female (57%). On average, mothers and fathers were in their early 40s with the parents' mean age of 43 (SD= 6.1) and a range of 28 to 61. The majority of parents in the study were Taiwanese (76%), high school graduates (35%), doing work as laborers or farmers (26%), married (91%), and Buddhist (50 %).

Demographic Description of the Children with DMD and Their Families

The age of the children ranged from 3-25 years (mean = 14.3, SD = 4.6). Twenty-three percent of the children were eighteen years old or more, and 41% were teenagers. Forty-six percent of the children could not raise their hand to their mouth, and 78% needed wheelchair assistance. Seventy-three percent of the children still attended school or received education at home (Table 3).

Sixty percent of families were living in an urban area, 76% were nuclear families, and 66% had an adolescent child. The majority of families had only one child (44%) and 42% had two children (Table 3).

Table 2

Demographic Characteristics of Parents for Current Study

Characteristics		No	%	
Gender	Male	54	42.9	
	Female	72	57.1	
Parent age	<=35 years	13	10.3	Mean age = 43 years
	36-40 years	28	22.2	SD = 6.1 years
	41-45 years	48	38.1	Range = 28-61 years
	>=46 years	27	21.4	
Ethnicity	Taiwanese	96	76.2	
	Chinese	13	10.3	
	Haika	15	11.9	
	Aboriginal	2	1.6	
Education	Elementary	153	11.9	
	Primary school	44	29.4	
	High school	16	34.9	
	College school	14	12.7	
	University or higher		11.1	
Occupation	Laborer of farmer	33	26.2	
	Technique	14	11.1	
	Government officer	13	10.3	
	Professional	12	9.5	
	Business	15	11.9	
	None or homemaker	39	31.0	
Marital status	Married	114	90.5	
	Separated	1	.8	
	Widowed	5	4.0	
	Divorced	3	2.4	
	Remarried	3	2.4	
Religion	Buddhism	63	50.0	
	Taoist	36	28.6	
	Christian	5	4.0	
	Catholic	1	.8	
	None	21	16.7	

Sample Size and Data Analysis

There were two types of statistical techniques, Pearson correlation and multiple regression, used to analyze the data. A power of .93 was reached with the sample of 126 subjects with an effect size of .3 and set alpha at .05 on the Pearson correlation. A power of .86 was reached with the sample of 126 subjects with an effect size of .15 and alpha set at .05 on the regression (Cohen, 1988).

Table 3

Demographic Characteristics of the Children with DMD and Families (N=80)

Characteristic		Frequency	%
Child age	Range = 3-25 years Mean =14.3 years SD = 4.6 years		
Child's upper extremity function	Can raise hand to mouth Can not raise hand to mouth	43 37	52.8 46.2
Child's lower extremity function	With wheelchair assistance Without wheelchair assistance	62 18	77.5 22.5
Child education in School or at home	Attended Not attended	58 22	72.5 27.5
Location	Rural Urban or Municipal	32 48	40.0 60.0
Family status	Nuclear Extended	61 19	76.3 23.8
Developmental stage of children in family	Preschool School Adolescent Adult	1 18 53 8	1.3 22.5 66.2 10.0
Sibling number	0 1 2 3	7 35 34 4	8.8 43.8 42.4 5.0

Procedure

Access to Study Population

The investigator contacted the leaders of KMU Hospital and the TMDA, the pediatric and adult neurologists, and the social worker of the TMDA to present the study and obtain permission to contact eligible participants. Permission was obtained (see letters of support, Appendix A-G).

Data Collection

Eligible subjects (parents of children with DMD) were mailed a letter by the TMDA or were invited by the neurologists to participate in the study. Then the investigator made a phone call to ask the subjects to participate in the study; if the subjects agreed to fill out the questionnaires the investigator sent each family a cover letter with two sets of questionnaires and informed consents, which outlined the purpose and procedures of the study and assurance of confidentiality. The letter further informed them that the investigator would respect their right to refuse to participate if they were in distress. It was once again emphasized to the participants that all their responses would be held in strictest confidence and locked in a file cabinet, and that only a number would be used for subject identification. A telephone number was included in case there were further questions or consultations.

Parent participants were instructed to individually answer the questionnaires separately and avoid discussion of the questions with others. Each subject took approximately 40 minutes to complete the questionnaires. Each subject received a phone call from the investigator within the first week after mailing the questionnaires and again two weeks later to remind him or her to complete and return them. The researcher enclosed a payment envelope, consent forms, and another set of forms if the subjects lost them. The researcher also offered assistance by phone to help them complete the questions, and later contacted them if the questionnaires were not completed. The instrument data was entered by the investigator and rechecked to prevent artificial errors and loss of the sample. The researcher used SPSS (version 11) to survey the data and conduct the analysis.

Instruments

The Demographic Sheet

The demographic sheet included information about the child's level of disability (using criteria from the Barthel Index-BI) and the age when the child was diagnosed with

DMD. Family resources included parent's age and education, ethnicity, employment status, marital status, family location, religion, family income, and family size.

Barthel Index

The BI is a 10-item instrument measuring disability in terms of a person's level of functional independence in personal activities of daily living (Mahoney & Barthel, 1965). The BI contained items about feeding, moving from wheelchair to bed and return, grooming, transferring to and from a toilet, bathing, walking on a level surface, going up and down stairs, dressing, and continence of bowels and bladder. It was rated by observation. The BI has been used to measure disability in both adults and children.

Item scores (based on different levels of independence: independent = 0; need help or major help = 5; independent, minor help, or continent = 10; maximum independent = 15) were summed up to generate a total score. There were two items on a two-point scale, six items on a three-point scale, and two items on a four-point scale (Appendix H). Scores on each rating form were added for an overall score, with higher scores indicating greater independence. The scores ranged from 0 (totally dependent) to 100 (fully independent). This study used Shah, Vanclay, and Cooper's (1989) suggestion that scores of 0-20 indicated total dependency, 21-60 indicated severe dependency, 61-90 indicated moderate dependency, 91-99 indicated slight dependency, and 100 indicated complete independence.

The BI is an ordinal rating scale. Each item was rated in terms of whether the child could perform the task independently, with some assistance, or was dependent on help based on observation. The scores for each of the items were summed to create a total score. The higher the score, the more independent the person was (Mahoney & Barthel, 1965).

Validity

Wade and Hewer (1987) reported validity correlations ranged from .73 to .77 with an index of motor ability for 976 stroke patients. Wylie and White (1964) and Wylie (1967) found that the BI correlated well with clinical judgment and predicted mortality or ability to be discharged to a less restrictive environment.

Reliability

The BI had evidence of reliability and validity (Collin, Wade, Davis, & Horne, 1988). Sherwood, Morris, Mor, et al. (1977) reported high alpha reliability ranging from .953 to .965 for three samples of hospital patients suggesting that the test was internally consistent as a measure of self-care activities. Shah et al. (1989) reported alpha internal consistency coefficients of .87 to .92 for the original scoring system and .90 to .93 for a revised scoring system. It was .88 in the current study.

Family Characteristics

The demographic questionnaire included parental education, ethnicity, family religion, family annually income, parental employment, satisfaction with medical care, sibling health, family structure, family size, family development stage, parental age, and family location. The demographic variables of employment and annual income were used to measure family characteristics.

The Duke Health Profile

The DUKE is a 17-item measure of adult health - related quality of life and functional health status. The 17 items are divided into 6 scales, measuring positive functional health and 5 scales measuring negative functional health. The six scales of functional health include: physical, mental, social, general, perceived health, and self-esteem; higher scores indicate better health-related quality of life (greater functional health). The five scales of negative functional health include: anxiety, depression, anxiety-depression, pain, and disability; higher scores indicated greater dysfunctional health (Parkerson, 2002).

The physical, mental, social, and perceived health scales and the disability scale are independent of each other in that none of their items are shared, whereas the other scales are not independent because they shared single or multiple items extracted from the independent scales. The DUKE consists of 10 summary scores: physical health (5 items), mental health (5 items), social health (5 items), perceived health (1 item), self-esteem (5 items), anxiety (6 items), depression (5 items), pain (1 item), perceived health (1 item), and disability (1 item). A general health score was obtained by combing averages of the first subscales. Some items contributed to several summary scores; for example, number 4, "I gave up too easily," contributed to the mental health, self-esteem, and depression scales. Responses were made on a three-point scale (see Appendix I for the rating scale). A total score was calculated based upon a summary of the 17 items score was the mean of the raw scores transformed from a scale of 0-2 to a scale of 0-100 (raw scores of 0, 1, and 2 become final scores of 0, 50, 100) (see Appendix I for the DUKE scores of procedures). The higher score indicated better health (Parkerson, 2002).

Validity

The DUKE obtained adequate validity by using the Family Strengths and Family Inventory of Life Events (Parkerson et al., 1991). The 7-item anxiety-depression subscale of the DUKE (DUKE-AD) had been used as an effective screener for DSM-III-R major anxiety and depression. Validity had been strongly supported for the instrument. Tsai et al. (1993) also showed that the subscale scores of the DUKE were significantly correlated with demographic and clinical variables. The predicted relationships among the DUKE score and clinical variables supported the construct validity of the DUKE. The DUKE had been found to have significant correlations with the Psychological Symptom Scale, Tseng's Depression Scale, Chinese Health Questionnaire, and Family APGAR to support convergent and discriminate validity.

Reliability

Reliability estimated for the DUKE is the following: most of multi-item scales had Cronbach's alpha reliability coefficients in the .60 and .70, while the single item scales had test-retest coefficients in the .40 and .50 (Parkerson, 2002). Tsai, Chang, and Tseng (1993) compared the Chinese version of the DUKE with 557 adult outpatients' and 323 adults seeking general health examinations; they found that one-week interval test-retest reliability for the DUKE was .51 to .85 and internal consistent Cronbach alpha was .49 to .70. The study found that internal consistent Cronbach alpha for the DUKE was .81; physical health was .60, mental health was .52, and social health was .69.

In addition, the DUKE had been used mostly for primary care patients, but also for normal medical students and insurance policyholders, and for patients with chronic lung disease, insulin-dependent diabetes, end-stage renal disease requiring hemodialysis, and cardiac and musculoskeletal disorders (Medical Outcome Trust, 2001). The DUKE had been translated into a Chinese version (Medical Outcome Trust, 2001).

Family APGAR

Smilkstein (1978) designed the FAPGAR to evaluate adult satisfaction with social support from the family. The components of FAPGAR include adaptation, partnership, growth, affection, and resolve. Adaptation is "utilization of intra and extra familial resources for problem solving when family equilibrium is stressed during a crisis" (p.1232). Partnership is "the sharing of decision making and nurturing responsibilities by family members" (p. 1232). Growth is "the physical and emotional maturation and self-fulfillment that is achieved by family members through mutual support and guidance" (p. 1232).

Affection is "the caring or loving relationship that exists among family members" (p. 1232). Resolve is "the commitment to devote time to other members of the family for physical and emotional nurturing. It also usually involves a decision to share wealth and space" (p. 1232).

The FAPGAR is a 5-item measure of perceived family support (Smilkstein, 1978). Each item allowed three responses (2 = almost always, 1 = some of the time, 0 = hardly ever) (Appendix J). The total scores range from 0 to 10 (low to high satisfaction with family support). Lower scores indicate more parental distress (Gardner et al., 2001). All items were summed for a total score.

Validity

Construct validity. A correlation of .64 was found between FAPGAR and a therapist's rating of family functioning of mental health outpatients. Good et al. (1979) noted a correlation of .80 with the Pless-Satterwhite Family Function Index ($r = .80$). Foulke, Reeb, Graham, and Zyzanski (1988) used 140 families to explore the relationship between the FAPGAR and the Family Adaptation and Cohesion Evaluation Scales (FACES). They found that FAPGAR is highly correlated with the Cohesion Scale of FACES ($r = .70$) and moderately correlated with the Adaptability Scale ($r = .59$) to support construct validity.

Criterion validity. Moos and Moos (1981) reported a correlation of .54 ($p = .01$) with the FACES III cohesion sub-scale, and a correlation of -.40 ($p. = .01$) with Family Environment Scale to support the criterion validity. The Family Disruption from Illness Scale (FDIS) correlated significantly in the expected direction with all measures of family functioning: Family APGAR, $r = -.23$ (Gragert & Ide, 2003). Gwyther, Bentz, Drossman, and Berolzheimer (1993) found that the FAPGAR failed to detect family dysfunction found by psychological interview, but there was a strong relationship with the Minnesota Multiphasic Personality Inventory (MMPI) for 198 patients: 58 irritable bowel syndrome patients (IBS), 67 IBS nonpatients, and 73 normal subjects.

Gardner et al. (2001) suggested that low scores on the FAPGAR might measure parental distress, reflecting parental depression. Chen, Chen, Hsu, and Lin (1980) reported that well-adjusted Taiwanese students (N=1164) had higher scores in each subscale of the FAPGAR than the maladjusted students (N=1377). They also found that adopted children had significantly lower FAPGAR scores than biological children, and separated students had significantly lower FAPGAR scores than those living with parents. Chen (1988) reported that there was a relationship between the stimuli that children (N=100) perceived as stressful in the hospital and their scores on the adaptation and partnership subscale of FAPGAR. Lee et al. (1992) found that low FAPGAR scores could independently predict depressive symptoms among 397 patients with active pulmonary TB and the FAPGAR was significantly related to those who received TB treatment.

Discriminant validity. FAPGAR scores of married graduate students were significantly higher than scores of community mental health clinic patients (Smilkstein, Ashworth, & Montano, 1982). Good, Smilksteine, Good, Shaffer and Arons (1979) found a significant difference between the FAPGAR scores of the psychiatric outpatients and healthy adults groups. In addition, Hilliard, Gjerde, and Parker (1986) found significant differences in the mean FAPGAR score (respondents rating five-Likert scale) between nonsymptomatic patients (mean = 38) and patients with suggestive symptoms (abdominal pain of uncertain etiology, urticaria, peptic ulcer, irritable bowel syndrome) or clear symptoms (anxiety, depression, suicide attempt, marital dysfunction) (mean = 32). The results supported discriminate validity. In terms of psychometric validity, they also found a false-negative rate for the FAPGAR (19%) (insensitivity to psychological problems).

Reliability

The instrument has obtained satisfactory reliability scoring, ranging from .80 to .89 (Gillis, Neuhaus, & Hauck, 1990; Kirkevold, Gortner, Berg, & Saltvold, 1996; Smilkstein et al., 1982). The Cronbach α was .80, a high internal consistency for a sample of 291 women and 238 men whose average age was 19.7 years (Smilkstein et al., 1982). Inter-item correlations ranged from .24 to .67, and the inter-spouse correlation for the FAPGAR was .67 (Good et al., 1979; Smilkstein et al., 1982). Moos and Moos (1981) reported an alpha coefficient of .84. Kirkevold, Gortner, Berg, and Saltvold (1996), and Good et al. (1979) noted a split-half reliability coefficient of .93. Two-week interval test-retest reliability was .83 among 100 Taiwanese students (Chen et al., 1980). The Cronbach α of this study was .89.

The Family APGAR has been used to screen for lack of family social support (Murphy et al., 1998). Several researchers used the FAPGAR to evaluate family relationship of HIV-1 infected patients (Lee, 1999; Lee, Chuang, & Shen, 1994; Lee & Lin, 1989), and cardiac inpatients (Lee, 1991). It has also been used to look at family relationships in terms of health status, neurosis, severe mental symptoms, and coping strategies. Further, it has been used in the study by Chen, et al. (1980) in Taiwan when the instrument was translated into Chinese.

Family Hardiness Index

The FHI was "developed to adapt the concept of individual hardiness to the family unit" and consists of three components: commitment, challenge, and control (McCubbin et al. 2001, p. 273). According to McCubbin et al. (2001), commitment represents "family sense of internal strengths, dependability, and ability to work together to manage the difficulties" (p. 277). Challenge means "family efforts to be innovative, active, and to experience new things and to learn" (family believes that hardship is normal for life to change) (p. 277). Finally, control is defined as the "family sense of being in control of family life rather than being shaped by outside events and the victim of circumstances" (is the tendency to believe and act in a way that influence the course of life's events) (p. 277).

The Index was a 20-item instrument with a four-point scale that was constructed to measure three components: commitment-8 items, challenge-6 items, and control-6 items (McCubbin, McCubbin, & Thompson, 1986). Scoring of the FHI is done by the summation of the chosen response, which represents the degree to which the personal agree with the statement at the present time (0=False, 1=Mostly false, 2= Mostly true, 3=True). Nine of the items must be revised in order to ensure they are positively directed (3=False, 2=Mostly false, 1= Mostly true, 0=True) (Appendix K). Items were summed for a total score in the present study. High score indicates greater levels of family hardiness.

Validity

The concurrent validity was measured by examining the relationship with various indices, validity coefficient ranging from .15 to .23 for coherence, flexibility, and stability (McCubbin et al., 2001). The FHI correlated with Family Time and Routines, .23 (McCubbin et al., 2001) and with FACES II, .22 (Olson, Potner, & Bell, 1982). Construct validity was verified by factor loading that was reported to be in the range of .52 to .85.

Svavarsdottir (1997), using a sample of families of young children with asthma, found that a sense of coherence and general well-being were positively correlated with family hardiness, indicating a higher sense of coherence ($r = .75$ for the mothers' score, $r = .73$ for the highest score of the parents, $r = .81$ for the mean of the parents' score, $r = .60$ for the fathers' score). Higher reported physical and emotional well-being correlated with higher family hardiness ($r= .70$ for the mothers' score, $r = .60$ for the fathers' score) and also suggested that family hardiness was also positively correlated with family adaptation ($r = .57$ for the parents' highest score, $r = .72$ for the mean of the parents).

Campbell and Demi (2000) investigated the relationship among emotional distress, grief, and family hardiness in 20 adult children of missing-in-action fathers. They found the FHI subscale, commitment and control, was negatively correlated with all three Bereavement Experience Questionnaire-Short Form (BEQ-24) subscales, and the BEQ-24 Existential Loss was negatively correlated with two of the FHI subscales, challenge and control.

Family hardiness has been noted as a key variable in influencing family adaptation and family well-being (McCubbin & McCubbin, 1991; Newby, 1996; Svavarsdottir, 1997). Svavarsdottir's (1997) study suggested that family hardiness could predict family adaptation and the well being of mothers and fathers caring for children with asthma. Leske (2003) did not find significant differences in family strengths of hardiness and family well being and adaptation for patients who had trauma after surgery. Leske et al. (1998) suggested that the only significant variable of hardiness (family strength) to influence family adaptation was problem-solving communication. Ladewig et al. (1992) indicated that family hardiness and coping played a more important role in relation to long-term outcomes than for initial response to a crisis event, supporting predictive validity.

Reliability

The overall internal reliability for the original study for the FHI is .82 with subscale reliabilities of .73 to .82 (Sawin & Harrigan, 1994). Subsequently, studies reported a reliability of .73 for caregivers' burden among family members caring for patients receiving chemotherapy (Carey, Oberst, McCubbin, & Hughes, 1991), .80 reliability for the families of children with developmental disabilities for the total FHI (Failla & Jones, 1991), and subscale reliabilities from .49 to .77 (Failla & Jones, 1991). For the three subscales, the internal reliabilities were .81, .80, and .65 (McCubbin et al., 2001). Kuo (2000) measured the Chinese Family Hardiness Index with preterm labor families (using Cronbach's alpha) with fathers reported at .81, and .77 for mothers. A test-retest study at one month of families dealing with a technology-dependent chronic illness was .94 (Carey et al., 1991). McCubbin et al. (2001) reported that test-retest reliability was .86. The Cronbach α of the study was .81. The subscale of commitment was .69, challenge was .62, and control was .56.

There was no normative data on the FHI, but the FHI has been used in various populations of the chronically ill, such as persons with cancer (Mellon & Northouse, 2001; Northouse et al., 2002), disability (Failla & Jones, 1991; Olsen et al., 1999), asthma (Svavarsdottir, 1997), arthritis (Lambert, Lambert, Klipple, & Mewshaw, 1990), and hemodialysis (White, Richter, Koeceritz, & Lee, 2002). A few studies focused on immigrants

(Kamya, 1997), and victims of political violence (Campbell & Demi, 2000; Khamis, 1998) and traumatic events (Ladewig & Jessee, 1992; Leske, 2000; Leske & Jiricka, 1998). Family hardiness has been studied in families of children with a cardiac condition and families who have a child with diabetes (H. I. McCubbin et al., 1996).

McMaster Family Assessment Device (FAD - 60 items)

The McMaster Model of Family Functioning (MMFF) is based on systems, role, and communication theories, and evolved from work with non-clinical families (Sawin & Harrigan, 1995). The model identified six dimensions: problem solving, communication, roles, affective responsiveness, affective involvement, and behavior control. Six of the scales on the FAD reflected the dimensions of family functioning outlined in the MMFF (Epstein, Bishop, & Levin, 1978). Additionally, Epstein, Baldwin, and Bishop (1983) selected the items most highly intercorrelated, which resulted in the creation of a general functioning dimension, which assessed overall health of the family.

Epstein et al. (2003) identified "family problem solving as a family ability to resolve problems to a level that maintains effective family functioning" (p. 587), "communication as the exchange of verbal information within a family" (p. 589), "family role as the repetitive patterns of behavior by which family members fulfill family functions" (p. 590), "affective responsiveness as the ability to respond to a given stimulus with an appropriate quality and quantity of feelings" (p. 594), "affective involvement as the family shows interest in and values the particular activities and invest themselves in one another" (p. 595), and "behavior control as the pattern a family adopts for handling behavior in three areas-physically dangerous situations, involving meeting and expressing drives and psychobiological needs, and interpersonal socializing behavior" (p. 596).

The present study used the FAD which consisted of 60 items (with seven items added to three of the scales to increase reliability of the original 53-item version) (Bernstein, Garbin, & McClellan, 1983). The scales and dimensions of the FAD included: 6 items for problem solving, 9 items for communication, 11 items for roles, 6 items for affective responsiveness, 7 items for affective involvement, 9 items for behavior control, and 12 items for general functioning. Epstein, Baldwin, & Bishop (1983) developed the FAD-3 in the United States. Responses are made on a four-point scale "strongly agree, agree, disagree, to strongly disagree." One total score ranging from 1 to 4, a lower score corresponds to greater health (Appendix L).

Validity

The construct validity of the FAD was appropriate (Browne, Arpin, Coey, Fitch, & Gafni, 1990). The FAD scores have been related to family function focused on parenting (McFarlane, Bellissimo, & Norman, 1995), psychological well-being (Byles, Bryne, Bolye, & Offord, 1988; Martin, Rozanes, Pearce, & Allison, 1995; Wenniger, Hageman, & Arrindell, 1993); and to the parent-child relationship scale (Wamboldt, Wamboldt, Gavin, & Mctaggart, 2001). Shek (2002) showed that the FAD scores were significantly correlated with measures of trait anxiety, existential well-being, life satisfaction, and sense of mastery. Kabacoff, Miller, Bishop, Epstein, and Keitner (1990) used oblique multiple group confirmatory factors analysis to show that over 90 % of the FAD items were loaded on factors hypothesized by the McMaster Model. These findings support the construct validity of the FAD. The predicted relationship between the scales of the FAD, FACES (96 items) and the Family Unit Inventory (FUI) provided adequate evidence of the concurrent validity for the FAD (Kabacoff, Miller, Bishop, Epstein, & Keitner, 1990; Van der Putten et al., 1999). The relationship between the FAD and FACES II, a revised version of FACES (30 items), did not correspond to theoretical predictions, but a more linear relationship was obtained.

The FAD was able to discriminate psychiatric patients and healthy employees or university students to support its discriminant validity (Epstein, Baldwin, & Bishop, 1983; Miller et al., 1985; Shek, 2002). Miller et al. (1985) used mean cutoff scores for each subscale, which ranged from 2.1 to 2.4, to discriminate between healthy and unhealthy families. It was able to discriminate between healthy families, and psychiatric families when compared to families rated by clinicians. Lampher (1999) found that students who were at high risk for suicide ideation scored significantly higher on the FAD, which suggested family dysfunction. Those data supported discriminative validity of the FAD. The FAD has been found to have low correlations with social desirability ($r = .06-.19$), moderate correlations with global measures of marital functioning such as the Dyadic Adjustment Scale ($r = .47$), and the Locke-Wallace Marital Satisfaction Scale ($r = .59$), and theoretically consistent correlations with other measures of family functioning (Miller et al., 1985). Keitner, et al. (1992) and Miller, et al. (1992) reported that the FAD was predictive of recovery from major depression.

Reliability

The FAD has been found to have high levels of internal consistency ranging from .72 to .92 across a variety of different types of families (Epstein et al., 1983), and acceptable levels of test-retest reliability ranging from .66 to .76 (Miller et al., 1985). Roncone and colleagues (1998) reported that test-retest reliability for the Italian FAD ranged from .69 to .91. Shek (2002) reported that test-retest for the Chinese secondary school students ranged from .52 to .81; and the alpha reliability was acceptable, ranging from .61 to .91 except for affective responsiveness (.44) and behavior control (.56). Chen (2002) reported that the acceptable alpha reliability of the Chinese FAD version ranged from .52 to .82, except for behavior control (.52). Wang and Phinney (1998) reported alpha reliability of .29 to .74 in the evaluation of immigrant Chinese and Anglo-American mothers. The Cronbach α of this study was .67 for problem solving, .81 for general function, .60 for communication, .62 for roles, .64 for affective involvement, .67 for affective responsiveness, and .36 for behavior control (Table 4).

Table 4

Internal Consistency Reliability of Measuring the Subscales of the Family Functioning Described in the Current Study (N=126)

	Number of Item	Alpha
Problem solving score	6	.67
Communication score	9	.60
General	12	.81
Role	11	.62
Affective responsiveness	6	.67
Affective involvement	7	.64
Behavior control	9	.36

The FAD has been used to assess family functioning in different countries such as Australia (Sawyer, Sarris, Baghurst, Cross, & Kalucy, 1988), Hungary (Keitner et al., 1991), Italy (Roncone et al., 1998), the Netherlands (Wenniger et al., 1993), the United Kingdom (Stevenson-Hinde & Akister, 1995), Hong Kong (Shek, 2002; Shek, Lai, & Lai, 1998), and Taiwan (Huang, 1994); and different populations with psychiatric disorders (Friedmann et al., 1997), anorexia nervosa (Gowers & North, 1999), depression (Keitner, 1990; Stein et al., 2000), cardiac rehabilitation (O'Farrell, Murray, & Hotz, 2000), psychopathology (Lieb et al.,

2000), traumatic brain injury (Max et al., 1998; Rivara et al., 1996), and adolescence (McFarlane et al., 1995).

The particular strength of the FAD is the number of languages in which the instrument is available, making it possible to study and compare families from a variety of cultures. Sawin et al. (1994) has recommended the FAD as a convenient, easy, and rapidly administered instrument that is useful in clinical and research settings to evaluate family functioning. It has been translated into twelve languages. Tutty (1995) reported that the FAD holds excellent psychometric properties.

Summary

Using a descriptive correlation study with a cross-sectional and predictive design, this quantitative research study explored factors associated with family functioning in families with a DMD child. One hundred and twenty-six parents with DMD children participated in the study. The participants answered four separated instruments that measured family health, family hardiness, family support, and family functioning and then a family demographic sheet that included the children's degree of disability. Instruments achieved appropriate alpha internal consistency coefficients. Sample size and power analysis were used for Pearson correlation and multiple regression, with a moderate effect and alpha = .05 selected.

RESULTS

This chapter will report factors associated with functioning among families who have DMD children. These factors included family health, family support, family hardiness, and age when diagnosed with DMD. The demographic characteristics of the subjects, DMD children, families; and the subscales of the instruments reliability were presented in the preceding chapter. The presentation of the results is organized by each aim of the study.

Data Analysis

Data were analyzed using SPSS (version 11.0) and AMOS (version 4.0). Internal consistency reliability using Cronbach's alpha coefficients ranged from 0.81 to .92 (Table 5), indicating high internal consistency reliability for the instruments used in the present study. Hierarchical multiple regression and path analysis were used to test the model.

Table 5

Measures of Central Tendency for Child Disability, Family Resources (Family Health, Family Hardiness, and Family Support), and Family Functioning

Empirical indicator (Instruments)	Items	Alpha	Range	Theoretical range	Mean	SD
Child disability (BI)	10	.88	10-100	0 - 100	38.65	25.40
Family health (DUKE)	17	.81	29.41 - 100	0 - 100	67.48	15.79
Family hardiness (FHI)	20	.81	20-58	0 - 60	41.24	7.70
Family support (FAPGAR)	5	.89	0-10	0 - 10	6.63	2.86
Family Functioning (FAD)	60	.92	1.43 - 2.63	1 - 4	2.10	.29

The specific aims for the study were as follow:

Aim 1: Describe the child's level of disability, access to care, and family characteristics

Children's level of disability and access to care. The age range of the children when diagnosed with DMD was 1-15 years (mean = 6.2, SD = 2.8), which indicated when the children began to have access to professional care (Table 6).

The total Barthel Index score of the children at the time of the study ranged from 10 to 100 (mean: 38.65, SD = 25.4) (Table 5). Thirty-eight (47.5%) of the DMD children had a rated score of 21-60, indicating severe dependency and twenty-eight (35%) of the DMD children had a rated score of 0-20, indicating total complete dependency (Table 6).

Family characteristics. Forty-four percent of the families reported annual income of less than $10,000 (NT$ 360,000); 10% were over $30,000 (NT$ 1,080,000). Low-income families were the majority in this study. Fifty-six percent of parents were employed and 44% were unemployed, retired, or homemakers (Table 6).

Aim 2: Describe for family health, family hardiness, family support, and family functioning

Normative data of family health. The total family health score rated by the individual parents ranged from 29-100 (mean: 67.5, SD = 15.8) with higher scores reflecting higher functional health (Table 5). Fifty-two percent of the parents reported a family health score greater than 67.7, indicating better health. Twenty-one percent of the parents reported a family health score lower than 55.9, indicating dysfunctional health. The higher the score the better the health. Therefore, most of the parent's (52%) reported that they were overall healthy.

Table 6

DMD Children's Disability and Access to Care, and Family Characteristics(N=80)

Characteristic		Frequency	%
Age when diagnosed with DMD	Range = 1-15 years Mean = 6.2 years SD = 2.8 years		
	Barthel Index score[a]		
Disability Level	0- 20	28	35.0
	21- 60	38	47.5
	61 -90	11	13.7
	>=91	3	3.8
Annually income[b]	<=10,000	35	43.8
	10,001 - 15,000	13	16.2
	15,001 - 20,000	14	17.5
	20,001 - 25,000	6	7.5
	25,001 - 30,000	4	5.0
	> 30,000	8	10.0
Employment	Employed	71	56.3
	Unemployed	5	4.0
	Retired or homemaker	50	39.7

[a] Total raw score <= 60 indicated severe dependency
 Total raw score>60 indicated mild dependency
[b] 1 US$ = 36 NT$

The mean scores and standard deviation of the subscales of family health are presented in Figure 3. The mean of physical, mental, and social health scores of the parents were 66.1

(SD = 19.5, range 20-100), 64.1 (SD = 19.7, range: 20-100), and 65.2 (SD = 21.2, range 10-100) respectively; six percent of the parents scored lower than 40 for the three subscales indicating poor physical, mental, and social health. Four percent of the parents scored lower than 40 (mean = 71.5, SD = 21.5, range 20-100) for the self-esteem subscale indicating impaired self-esteem. Twelve percent of the parents scored lower than 50.0 for the perceived health (mean = 78.2, SD = 34.9, range 0-100) indicating impaired perceived health. Eight percent of the parents scored higher than 50.0 for the pain (mean = 43.3, SD = 26.3, range 0-100) indicating current pain. Eight percent of the parents scored higher than 50.0 for the disability (mean = 7.9, SD = 19.4,

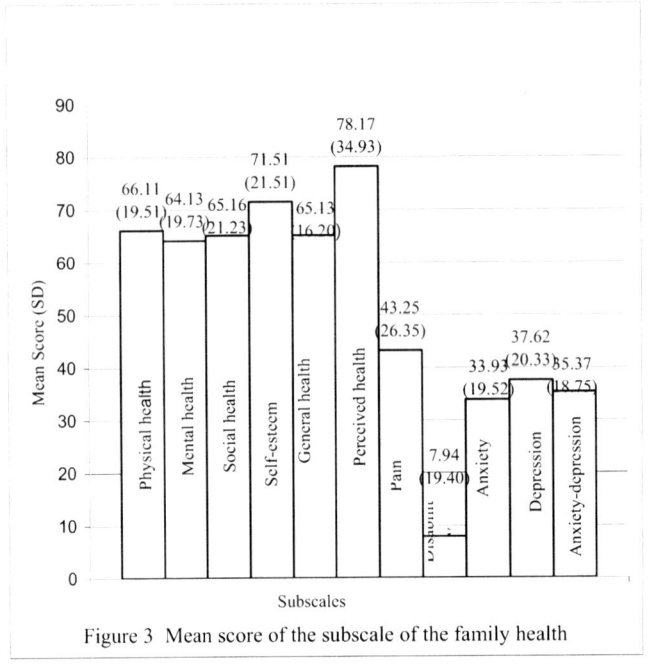

Figure 3 Mean score of the subscale of the family health

range 0-100) indicating disability. Nine percent of the parents scored higher than 58.3 (mean = 33.9, SD = 19.5, range 0-88.33) indicating anxiety. Seven percent of the parents scored higher than 60 (mean = 37.6, SD = 20.3, range 0-90) indicating depression. Nine percent of the parents scored higher than 57.1 (mean = 35.4, SD = 18.8, range 0–85.72) indicating anxiety-depression.

Normative Data of Family Hardiness. The ranged obtained on the total family hardiness scale (FHI) was: 20-58 (mean = 41.2, SD = 7.7) with higher scores reflecting greater hardiness (Table 5). The majority of families reported high hardiness scores (49%), indicating a hardier family, and ten percent of the parents scored less than 32 indicating a weaker family.

Three subscales of family hardiness are presented in Figure 4. The mean of the commitment score was 18.22 (SD = 3.62, range 6-24), seven percent of the parents scored lower than 13 indicating low commitment. Eight percent of the parents scored less than 8 on the challenge subscale (mean = 11.57, SD = 3.1, range 0-18), indicating a low degree of challenge. Five of the parents scored less than 7 on control (mean = 11.38, SD = 3.0, range 4-17), indicating a low sense of control.

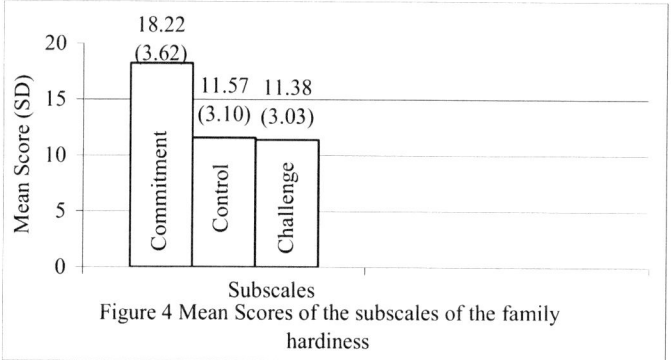

Figure 4 Mean Scores of the subscales of the family hardiness

Normative Data of Family Support. The range obtained on the total family support (FAPGAR) was 0-10 (mean = 6.63, SD = 2.9) with higher scores reflecting more support (Table 5). Over 50% of the parents scored higher than 6, indicating greater family support; 35% of the parents scored less than 6 indicating lower family support.

The mean and standard deviation of the five subscales of family support are shown in Figure 5. Sixteen percent of the subjects scored less than 1 on adaptability, indicating that they lacked the utilization of resources to solve problems; nineteen percent scored less than 1 on partnership, indicating the lack of sharing of decision making and nurturing responsibilities. Thirteen percent scored less than 1 on growth, indicating their lack of emotional maturation and self-fulfillment; ten percent scored less than 1 on affective, indicating their lack of a caring and loving relationship, and eight percent scored less than 1 on resolve indicating the lack of commitment to devote time to other family members.

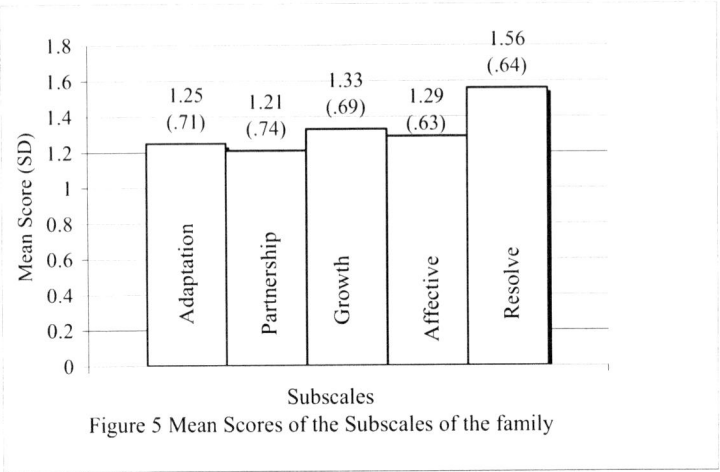

Figure 5 Mean Scores of the Subscales of the family

Normative Data of Family Functioning. The total family functioning scores on the FAD ranged from 1.43 to 2.63 (mean = 2.10, SD = .29) (Table 5). Nine percent of the parents scored higher than 2.46, indicating family dysfunction, and 48 % of the parents scored lower than 2.14, indicating positive functioning.

Seven subscales of the FAD are presented in Figure 6. The mean of problem solving was 1.95 (SD = .39, range 1.0-3.67). Ten percent of the parents scored higher than 2.33, indicating worse problem solving, and 45 % of the parents scored less than 2.0, indicating positive problem solving. Four percent of the parents scored higher than 2.56 on communication (mean = 2.11, SD = .35, range 1.0-3.11), indicating worse communication, and 37% scored less than 2.11, indicating positive communication. Six percent of the parents scored higher than 2.64 on role (mean = 2.22, SD = .33, range 1.36-3.18), indicating worse role functioning, and 46% scored less than 2.18, indicating positive role functioning. Ten percent of the parents scored higher than 2.50 on affective

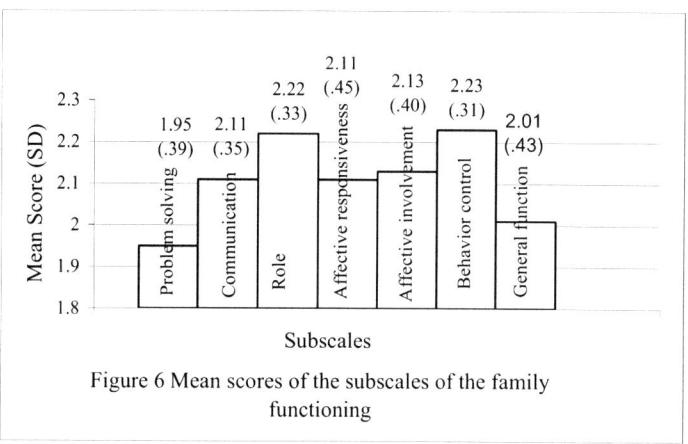

Figure 6 Mean scores of the subscales of the family functioning

responsiveness (mean = 2.11, SD = .45, range 1.0-3.67), indicating worse affective responsiveness, and 35% scored less than 2.17, indicating positive affective responsiveness. Four percent of the parents scored higher than 2.71 on affective involvement (mean = 2.13, SD = .40, range 1.14-3.14), indicating less affective involvement, and 44 % scored less than 2.14, indicating more affective involvement. Six percent of the parents scored higher than 2.67 on behavior control (mean = 2.23, SD = .31, range 1.44-3.0), indicating worse behavior control, and 42% scored less than 2.11, indicating better behavior control. Six percent of the parents scored higher than 2.58 on general functioning (mean = 2.01, SD = .43, range 1.08-3.17), indicating worse general functioning, and 46% scored less than 2.0, indicating better general functioning.

Aim 3: Describe the relationship among child's disability and access to care (age when diagnosed with DMD), family resources (family characteristics, family health, family support, family hardiness), and family functioning

Pearson correlation coefficients were used with interval data and with non-numeric data with dummy variables or dummy coding to explore what factors were associated with family functioning. A correlation matrix among child's disability and access to care, family resources, and family functioning appears in Table 7.

Correlation between child disability and access to care and family functioning. From the correlational analysis, the family functioning score had a significantly small positive correlation with age when diagnosed with DMD (r = .20, p = .02), but was not significantly correlated with child's dependency level (r = .06, p = .52) (Table 7). Detecting the disease early increased family functioning.

  Correlation between family characteristics and family functioning. Table 7 shows that the family functioning score has no significant correlation with family annual income (r = .17, p = .06) and parents' employment (r = -.06, p = .48) (Table 7). The results indicate that family annual income and parents' employment were not correlated with family functioning.

Table 7

Intercorrelation Among Child Disability and Access to Care, Family Resources,

and Family Functioning

Variable	1	2	3	4	5	6	7
1 Age when diagnosed of DMD	1.00						
2 Child disability (dependency)	-.22*	1.00					
3 Annual income	.26**	-.13	1.00				
4 Employment	-.09	.07	-.27**	1.00			
5 Family hardiness [a]	-.21*	.11	-.16	.05	1.00		
6 Family health [a]	.01	-.05	-.06	.19*	.51**	1.00	
7 Family support [a]	-.01	-.08	-.10	.13	.55**	.53**	1.00
8 Family functioning [b]	.20*	.06	.17	-.06	-.74**	-.60**	-.66**

** Correlation is significant at the 0.01 level (2-tailed).

* Correlation is significant at the 0.05 level (2-tailed).

[a] Higher score is higher, better, or greater

[b] Lower score is better

  Correlation of family hardiness, family health, family support, and family functioning. Table 7 also shows that family functioning had significantly high negative correlation with family hardiness (r = -.74, p = .00), and moderate negative correlation with family health (r = -.60, p = .00) and family support (r = -.66, p = .00). The higher the score of family functioning is, the lower the score on the family hardiness, family health, and family support. The family functioning score is a reverse score. Therefore, healthy family functioning was associated with higher family hardiness, greater family support, and better family health.

The variance shared between family functioning and family hardiness was 55% (95% CI for r = .643-.804). The variance shared between family functioning and family health was 36% (95% CI for r = .475-.701). The variance shared between family functioning and family support was 44% (95% CI for r = .597-.783). In other words, the independent variables- family hardiness, family health, and family support- were significant variables accounting for 55%, 36%, and 44% of variance in family functioning, respectively.

In addition, family hardiness had a significantly moderate positive correlation with family health (r = .51, p = .00) and family support (r = .55, p = .00); family health had a significantly moderate positive correlation with family support (r = .53, p = .00). Family hardiness accounted for 26% of the variance of family health (95% CI for r = .383-.639). Family support accounted for 30% of the variance of family hardiness (95% CI for r = .432-.677). Family support accounted for 28% of the variance of family health (95% CI for r = .384-.643).

The high or moderate negative correlation coefficients among the independent variables of family health (r = -.60), family support (r= -.66), and family hardiness (r = -.74) with family functioning suggest the absence of multicollinearity. Indications of multicollinearity are high correlations between independent variables (> .80); if correlations are above .95, there are serious problems (Glantz & Slinker, 1990). These higher negative associations indicated that parents with higher family hardiness, family health, and family support scores reported lower family function scores (meaning healthier family functioning).

Correlation between child disability, access to care, and family resources.
Table 7 shows that there were no significant correlations between child disability and family annual income, parents' employment, family hardiness, family health, family support, or family functioning. Age when diagnosed with DMD was significantly correlated with family hardiness (r = -.21, p = .02) and family annual income (r = .26, p = .003) but not significantly correlated with family health (r = .01, p = .88) or family support (r = -.01, p = .94) (Table 7). The variance shared between family hardiness and access to care (age when diagnosed with DMD) was 4% (95% CI for r = .037-.361). Access to care accounted for 7% of the variance of family annual income (95% of CI for r = .094-.418).

Correlation between family characteristics and family resources. The correlation of parents' employment with family annual income (r = -.27, p = .002) and family health (r = .19, p = .04) was significantly low (Table 7). However, these three variables were correlated with each other. The results reflect that parents working fulltime report a healthier family when the annual income is over $15,000.

Aim 4: Determine how the child's level of disability and access to care, family health, family characteristics, family support, and family hardiness predict family functioning

The relationships among the child's disability (dependence) and access to care (age when diagnosed with DMD), family resources (family characteristics, family health, family support, and family hardiness), and family functioning were determined in two ways. First, the Pearson correlation coefficient (dummy coding was applied to transform category data to 0 and 1) was used with significance determined at the .05 level, and second a hierarchical multiple regression procedure was used with significance determined at the .05 level.

In order to determine each predictor variable with the best parameter possible, numeric data (parents' employment and family annual income) were converted to dummy coding (employment coding 1 = employed, 0 = unemployed); family annual income was coded as 1 = < $15,000, 0 > $15,000); furthermore, the raw score of the Barthel Index was coded as 1 > 60 to represent mild dependence and 0 <= 60 to indicate severe dependence. There were several statistical assumptions to investigate prior to doing the multiple regressions. The assumptions to examine were normality, homoscedasticity (equal variance), linearity, and independence of individual variables and the residuals (Hair, Anderson, Tatham, & Black, 1998).

For each value of the independent variable, the distribution of the dependent variable, family functioning, was normal distribution. The variance of the distribution of family functioning was constant for all values of the independent variables-family hardiness, family health, and family support. The relationship between family functioning and each independent variable was linear, and all observations were independent.

To examine scatterplots and normal probability plots of the residuals of the dependent variable, family functioning, and independent variables, family hardiness, family health, or family support, the assumption of normal distribution with constant variance held; the residuals of family functioning plotted against any independent variable, family hardiness, family health, or family support fell in a band centered around zero with a constant width (null plot) produced a straight line, so the data presented was consistent with the regression model (Glantz & Slinker, 1990; Hair et al., 1998). The residuals were homoscedasticity and normally distributed about the plane regression line.

In partial regression plots for each independent variable, the equation showed that the relationship of the dependent variable, family functioning, to the independent variable, family hardiness, family health, and family support, were linear. The absence of curvilinear relationships had a significant effect in the regression equation, both in slope and scatter of the points, which were demonstrated in partial plots of the dependent and independent variables in the present study.

All predictive variables were entered in regression analysis and detected multicollinearity. The results fit the assumption of collinearity by the condition index (CI) of each variable that was lower than 30. There were no more than two predictors with coefficient variances over .5; all correlation coefficients less were than .75 and the variance inflation factor (VIF) value of each variable was never over 2 (Table 7 & Table 8). No high multicollinearity evidence can avoid redundant information in the independent variables taken as a whole and a decrease in two variables happens to contain the same information (Glantz & Slinker, 1990).

Based on the theoretical model and the unique contribution of individual predictors on the criterion variable, all variables were significant determinants of family functioning: the total variance of explanation (R^2), R^2 change, and part correlations in the criterion variable among the cluster of variables having significantly (F value) entered in the hierarchical multiple regressions.

Hierarchical regression analysis on family functioning. Hierarchical multiple regression analysis (Table 10) was performed for the first block with all three family resource clusters entered into the equation model. These were family hardiness, family health, and family support (multiple R = .743 for the predictive variable of family hardiness on family functioning, .802 for adding the second variable of family health, and .817 for adding the third predictive variable of family support, all with/at a p = .00).

The level of accurate prediction is the coefficient of determinants R^2, compared to the simple regression model value of $.743^2$ or .5520, which uses only family hardiness; when family health is added to the regression analysis, R^2 increase to $.802^2$ or .6432. The means inclusion of family health in the regression analysis increases the prediction by 9.08 %. When family support is added to the regression analysis, R^2 increases to $.817^2$ or .6675, which increases the prediction by 2.42 %.

The first block, which contained family hardiness, family support, and family health, was significant and accounted for 66.8% of the variance in family functioning. This indicated that a higher family hardiness score, higher family support score, and more healthier parents were related to lower family functioning score (meaning better family functioning). In the second block, the child's level of disability and access to care variables resulted in the entry age when diagnosed with DMD. The child's disability did not enter the equation. The age when diagnosed with DMD (multiple R = .824, p = .00) showed significant bivariate correlation with family functioning. The age when diagnosed with DMD was entered in the equation, the added R^2 changed to .011, and the R^2 was .679. The second predictor accounted for 1.1 % of variance in family functioning after controlling for the first three predictors. The age when diagnosed with DMD was related to family functioning, indicating that an earlier diagnosis of DMD led to earlier access to professional care that was related to lower family functioning scores (meaning better family functioning).

In the third block of variables, none of the two family characteristics entered the model. As a result of the shared variance, the variable (multiple R= .824, p= .00) significantly correlated family functioning in the final regression model, including three family resources clusters and one disabled child and access to care cluster that explained 67.9 % of the variance in family functioning. About 67.9 % of the variance in the criterion variable family functioning was explained by first family hardiness, family health, and family support (66.8%), and second by age when diagnosed with DMD (1.1%). All results came out to be significant. The change R^2 was also significant for the second step (F = 64.08, df = 4, 121, p = .00). According to the data of part cor (squared semi-partial)-sr, the total variance explained by the four independent variables is a unique variance explained (part cor^2-sr^2) by family hardiness .1156, family health .0289, family support .0557, and age when diagnosed with DMD .0112.

The overall equation for predicting family functioning was:

Family functioning = 3.17– .02 (family hardiness)- .004 (family health)– .03 (family support)+ .01 (age when diagnosed of DMD). The final regression statistics for the full model was significant (R = .824, F $_{(4, 121)}$ = 64.08, p = .00).

Aim 5: Test the model of family stressors, resources, and functioning

In the initial path analysis, standardized beta coefficients indicated that family hardiness, family support, family health, and age when diagnosed with DMD were the independent predictors in the regression equations on family functioning. In addition, family health and family support were predictors in the regression on family hardiness, and family health was a predictor in the regression on family support. However, the age when diagnosed with DMD was not a predictor in the regression on family health and family support. The path analysis was not a good fit for the model (x^2 = 0, df = 0, RMSEA = .44). The model that was tested was drawn with the path analysis in figure 7. The standardized regression coefficient (beta) was used to examine the total effect of family resources (family

Table 8

Hierarchical Multiple Regression for Family Stress with Family Resources on Dependent Variable Family Functioning (N=126)

Model		R	R^2	Adjust R^2	F	B	SE	Beta	T	Part cor (sr)	VIF
1	(Constant)	.817	.668	.660	81.82***	3.27	.088		37.217***		
					(df=3,122)						
	Family hardiness					-.020	.002	-.482	-7.316***	-.382	1.593
	Family health					-.004	.001	-.198	-3.306**	-.160	1.536
	Family support					-.030	.007	-.290	-4.366***	-.228	1.625
2	(Constant)	.824	.679	.669	64.08***	3.17	.100		31.807***		
					(df=4,121)						
	Family hardiness					-.020	.002	-.445	-6.599***	-.340	1.713
	Family health					-.004	.001	-.212	-3.304**	-.170	1.554
	Family support					-.030	.007	-.303	-4.592***	-.236	1.638
	Diagnosed age					.011	.005	.110	2.066*	.106	1.076

*P<.05, **p<.01, ***p<.001

hardiness, family health, and family support), and family stressors (age when diagnosed with DMD), which had both direct and indirect effects on family functioning. The standardized regression coefficient (path coefficient) may be used to decompose the correlation in the model into direct and indirect effects, corresponding to direct and indirect paths reflected in the arrows in the model. This is based on the rules of a linear system. The total causal effect of variable i on j is the sum of the values of all the paths from i to j (Norris, 2001).

Considering "family functioning" as the dependent variable in the model and the independent variables -age when diagnosed with DMD, family hardiness, family health, and family support, the indirect effect was calculated by multiplying the path coefficients for each path from each independent variable oneself to family functioning. The path coefficients suggest that family hardiness (beta = -.45, p = .00), family support (beta = -.30, p = .00), and family health (beta = -.21, p = .001) were directly predicted to have a positive effect on family functioning. The direct effect of age when diagnosed with DMD (beta = .11, p = .04) was also directly predicted to have a positive effect on family functioning. There was an indirect effect of age when diagnosed with DMD on family functioning by two paths (a) family hardiness, indicated by – .21 x (- .45) or .0945,

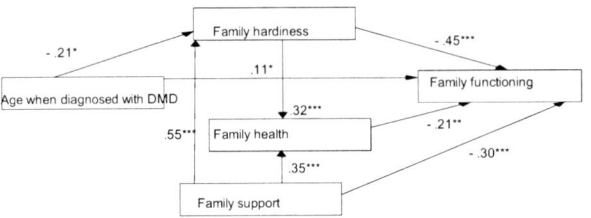

Figure 7 Final path analysis: influence of child disability, access to care, and, family resources on change in family functioning (standard beta weights are shown that include three regression equation models) * p < .05, ** p < .01, *** p < .001, Chi-squire = 1.413 df=2, p = .493, CMIN = 1.413, GFI =.996, AGFI = .966, NFI = .994, RFI= .976, RMSEA = .000
Model 1: Family hardiness, family health, family support, and age when diagnosed with DMD are predictors accounting for 68% of the variance of family functioning.
Model 2: Family hardiness and family support are predictors accounting for 35% of the variance of family health.
Model 3: Family support and age when diagnosed with DMD are predictors accounting 34.5% of the variance of the family hardiness.

and (b) family hardiness through family health, indicated by - .21 x .32 x (-.21) or .0141. The indirect effect of family hardiness on family functioning via family health was .32 x (-.21) or - .0672. The indirect effect of family support on family functioning was - .3579 via three paths (a) family heath, indicated by.35 x (-.21) or - .0735, (b) family hardiness, indicated by .55 x (-

.45) or - .2475, and (c) family hardiness through family health, indicated by .55 x .32 x (-.21)
or - .0369. There was no indirect effect of family health on family functioning.

In sum, the standardized total effect on family functioning by age when first diagnosed
with DMD was .22, family hardiness was - .52, family health was - .21, and family support
was - .66 (See Figure 7 or Table 9). Forty-three percent (.0945/.22) of the effect of early
disease diagnosis on family functioning was under the influence of family hardiness and 6.4%
(.0141/.22) was under the influence of family hardiness through family health; 50% (.11/.22)
of the total effect was mediated. By this computation of the total effect of family hardiness on
family functioning, 13.5% (- .0672 /- .52) of the total

Table 9

Standardized Direct and Indirect Effects for Family Stressors, Family
Resources on Family Functioning, Family Hardiness and Family Health

Dependent variable	Independent variable			
	Age when diagnosed with DMD	Family hardiness	Family health	Family support
Family functioning				
Total	.22	-.52	-.21	-.66
Direct	.11	-.45	-.21	-.30
Indirect	.11	-.07		-.36
Family health				
Total	-.07	.32		.53
Direct	----	.32		35
Indirect	-.07			.18
Family hardiness				
Total	-.21			.55
Direct	-.21			.55

effect was mediated by family health. Eleven percent (-.0735/- .66) of the effect of family
support on family functioning was under the influence of family health, 37.9% (- .2475/.66)
was under the influence of family hardiness, and 5.6% (- .0369/-.66) was under the influence
of family hardiness through family health. Fifty-four percent (-.3579/- .66) of the total effect
of family support on family functioning, -.3579, was mediated by family health, family
hardiness, and combining family hardiness with family health.

In addition, the direct effect of age when diagnosed with DMD (beta = -.21, p = .02)
was predicted to have a negative effect on family hardiness. The path coefficients indicating
the standardized direct effects, as well as the standardized total effect of age when diagnosed

with DMD on family hardiness was -.21. The standardized direct effect, as well as the standardized total effect of family support on family hardiness, was .55. The standardized direct effect, as well as the standardized total effect of family hardiness on family health was .32. Path analysis decomposed total effect of family support on family health (.53) into direct effect of family support on family health (.35) and the effect of family support that was indirect through family hardiness (.18). The standardized indirect effect, as well as the standardized total effect of age when diagnosed with DMD through family hardiness on family health, was - .07 (see Table 9).

Conclusion

The researcher used path analysis to test a model of the effects of family resources and child disability and access to care on family functioning in families with DMD children. A higher score on the perceived health measure indicated a higher level of positive health and a lower level of negative health. A higher score of family support indicated higher support to the DMD family. A higher score of family hardiness indicated greater levels of family hardiness. A higher score of family functioning indicated lower levels of family functioning. Results of hierarchical regression analysis of possible predictors of family functioning in a sample of 126 parents with DMD children showed higher scores of family hardiness, family health, and family support; earlier diagnosis of DMD was associated with healthier family functioning (lower score of family functioning) and higher family hardiness. The parents who reported higher scores of family hardiness and family support were associated with better health. Results of the path analysis revealed that family hardiness, family health, family support, and age when diagnosed with DMD accounted for 68% of the variance of family functioning; family hardiness and family support accounted for 35% of the variance of family health; and family support and age when diagnosed with DMD accounted for 34.5% of the variance of family hardiness.

DISCUSSION

Based on the results from this study of parents of children with DMD, the major components of the Conceptual Model of Family Stressors, Resources, and Functioning were supported. In this chapter, the findings of the study will be discussed, first by examining the major concepts and variables in the context of findings from other studies, followed by the implications of the major findings from this study.

Family Stressors, Resources, and Functioning Status

Family Stressors

The age of the child's diagnosis with DMD varied from 1 to 15 years. Because one-third of the children were diagnosed late, their access to professional care was limited. Eighty-three percent of families needed to completely assist with their daily activities. Families who received accurate information about the disease too late had difficultly coping with the chronic disability. Overload and uncertainty caused families much stress.

Family Resources

Family health. These parents had less physical, mental, and social health; lower self-esteem and perceived their health poorer than middle age female and male policyholders of a health insurance company (Parkerson, 2002). Except for physical health, the parents reported lower scores on all positive health subscales compared with 50-65 year old policyholders (Parkerson, 2002). They also reported more anxiety, depression, pain, and disability (Parkerson, 2002). Nereo et al. (2003) found that mothers of children with DMD have higher stress than a normative group because of problem behaviors of children with DMD, especially in social interactions (Nereo et al., 2003). These findings suggest that the parents in this study may have had more tension and poorer health status. The parents not only had physical overload because of caring for the children who needed complete assistance, but they also experience anxiety and depression because of their children's behavior problems and the progressive, and life-threatening nature of DMD.

Family hardiness. The mean of family hardiness for 126 parents with DMD children was less than the mean of mothers and fathers with young children of asthma; mothers and fathers of children with cardiac conditions; and mothers and fathers of children with diabetes (McCubbin et al., 2001). These differences between children with DMD and other difficult conditions in different cultures should be explored, as well as the differences in the mean scores in different diseases or phenomenon within the same country. Less than 50% of the families in the study were hardy; families with lower hardiness scores had difficulty finding resources, were anxious or depressed, and had health problems.

Family Support

Parents in this study had lower scores of family support than did families with and without other chronic conditions reported in the literature (Gwyther et al., 1993). Thirty-five percent of the parents in the study scored lower than 6 on the FAPGAR, a higher rate than Smucker, Wildman, Lynch, and Revolinsky's (1995) study, which found that only 15 % of families with well children score this low. Furthermore, Gardner's et al (2001) found that 31% of families with a child having psychosocial problems scored below 6 on the FAPGAR.

Family Functioning

For every dimension except behavior control, these parents had better functioning than clinician-rated healthy and unhealthy families; but communication score and affective involvement were worse than the healthy group (Miller et al., 1985). Hawley's (2000) study emphasized that inability to communicate was the major obstacle to family functioning. And in the early stage, several scholars have utilized communication in their research framework (Epstein et al., 1978; Olson et al., 1979). Psychiatric families had a significantly higher score on all the FAD subscale scores except behavior control (Miller et al., 1985). Chen and Liu (1989) reported that there were differences associated with problem solving, communication, role, affective involvement, behavior control, and general function between normal families and psychiatric patients' families.

Relationships Among Family Stressors, Resources, and Functioning

Family Stressors, Family Resources, and Family Functioning

Overall, of all the major variables investigated in this study, earlier detection of DMD, and higher scores on family hardiness, family health, and family support were associated with better family functioning. This suggests that early diagnosis of DMD in children may provide early access to professional care and the resources parents need to adapt and function well. It may be, however, that highly functioning families are more likely to seek on encourage evaluation of their child's grass motor delay sooner than families with poorer functioning, a possibility this study did not address, given its cross-sectional design.

The child's disability level was not significantly correlated with family functioning, family hardiness, family support, or family health. While this finding was surprising, others have found that higher family functioning was not related to the child's disability status (Kim, 2002; Olsen et al., 1999); whereas others reported an inverse relation between family functioning and severity of adolescent's and young adult's injury or disability status (Magill-Evans et al., 2001). Failla et al. (1991) found that mothers who had a developmentally disabled child showed a significantly positive relationship between family hardiness and family functioning; and between family hardiness and coping behavior, which are related to strengthening the relationships within the family. The present study did not find that the degree of the child's disability was positively related to family hardiness, family support, and family health. This may have been due to an increasing awareness and knowledge of the children's condition, and unlimited access to healthcare. The significant relationship between child health, family health, and family functioning has been found in other studies (Shek, 2002; Wells & Whittington, 1993) and reinforces the notion that the promotion of child health is central to all interventions in families with DMD children.

In addition, a strong positive correlation among family hardiness, family health, family support, and healthy family functioning suggests evidence of construct validity or criterion validity of family functioning. Bristol (1987) and Bennet and DeLuca (1996) reported that support from significant others and social support has a positive affect on family functioning. Wu and Huang (1997) reported that there was a significant relationship between family functioning and expressed emotion for the caregivers of family members with psychiatric conditions. Heru and Ryan (2003) found that family functioning and depression were closely associated with the caregivers of patients with chronic or recurrent mood disorders. The findings from this study suggest that lower family functioning was associated with less family hardiness and worse psychological health, which in turn was associated with less family support and a later age of diagnosis with DMD.

Family Characteristics, Family Hardiness, Family Support, and Family Health

The socioeconomic factors of family annual income and parents' employment were not found significantly related to family functioning. These may not have been the best parameters to assess because of centering the same classification of the sample. These findings are similar to previous studies in that none of the family characteristics have been found to be associated with family functioning (Lieb et al., 2000; Merikangas, Avenevoli, Dierker, & Grillon, 1999). However, parental education, number of children, severity of the child's condition, and the child's diagnosis have been found to correlate significantly with family hardiness, social support, stress, and coping (Huang, 1996).

The significant correlation between family support and family hardiness found in this study supports Olsen et al. (1999) and McCubbin et al. (1996) who found that family support was positively correlated with family hardiness. However, there was no evidence that income was related to family hardiness and family support. The DMD children from families with low annual income and low level of employment rate in this study were eligible to receive government support for special education, rehabilitation, and other specialized care. This may have contributed to their resiliency.

Determining the Predictive Variables Effect on Dependent Variable

Predictive Variables Effect on Family Functioning

Family stressors. The *child's disability level* did not enter the equation model of Family Stressors, Resources, and Functioning, which indicated that the child's disability level was not a significant predictor of family functioning. The child disability was not associated with family hardiness, family health, and family support. The level of dependency of the child did not significantly enter the equation of hierarchical multiple regressions on the family functioning. One explanation for this finding is that by the time of the study parents had already adjusted to their child's diagnosis, making it possible for them to develop healthy family communication and a positive parenting style.

Access to care was a significant positive predictor of family functioning, suggesting that early detection of the disease may have allowed the family access to needed services and support. Fifty percent of the total effect of access to care was an indirect effect on family functioning. This result suggests that both family hardiness and family hardiness combined with family health, is an important mediator for access to care on family functioning.

Family characteristics. Sociodemographic variables were found to play an unimportant role in explaining the dependent variable, family functioning, in the study. Of the family demographic characteristic domains, parents' employment and family annual income in this study were not consistent with other studies which found that income was negatively related to family functioning or well-being (Friedmann et al., 1997). The other characteristics were not considered in this study because the sample size was not large enough to use more than eight variables so the results could not be inferred and generalized (Hair et al., 1998; Thorndike, 1978). The low level of income reported from respondents may have skewed the results of the study than if the sample was more representative of the general population. However, all the children in this study had insurance coverage for their DMD-related health care.

Family health. The findings in this study were consistent with other studies which found that family health or psychological morbidity was directly or indirectly related to family functioning (Magill-Evans et al., 2001), but was not support most studies' finding that severity of child disease was related to family functioning (Fornari et al., 1999; Gowers & North, 1999; King et al., 1993; Luescher et al., 1999; Pal et al., 2002; Stein et al., 2000; Tamplin & Goodyer, 2001; Tamplin et al., 1998). In this study family health only directly affected family functioning; there was no indirect effect on family functioning. Family health contributed to a small percent of unit variance explaining family functioning. But family health was a mediating factor for family hardiness, family support, and access to care in their effects on family functioning (see figure 7).

This study did not explore the effect of subscales of family health on family functioning. Stein's (2000) findings that fathers of children with major depression scored significantly lower on the FAD scales of behavioral control and general functioning, compared to the fathers of other high-risk children; and mothers of high-risk children had significantly lower scores on the roles and affective involvement dimensions of the FAD compared with mothers of low-risk children. Heru and Ryan (2003) found that family functioning and depression were closely associated with the caregivers of patients with chronic or recurrent mood disorders.

Family hardiness. Huang (1996) found that family hardiness was a stronger predictor of family stress, coping, and family functioning than social support in families of children with developmental disability. Failla et al. (1991) found that family hardiness, family stressors, and functional support could predict the mothers' satisfaction with family functioning. They suggested that family hardiness could diminish the effects of stress, increase the use of support, and facilitate adaptation.

Results of this study suggest that the desirable outcome -family functioning- is associated with family hardiness, and that family hardiness mediated family functioning through age when diagnosed with DMD are important findings. One explanation of these findings is that parents' experience with difficult challenges at an earlier time in their family's life may have resulted in parents who were stronger and more resilient because of access to professional care or because they were already hardy prior to their child's diagnosis. Family hardiness was the major mediating factor for age when diagnosed with DMD and the effect of family support on family functioning. Family health was a mediating factor for family hardiness on family functioning (see Figure 7).

Hardy people have a tendency to see life events as less stressful than others, an ability to cope more effectively with stressful events, and a more conscientious approach to health care. The results suggest that psychosocial interventions that focus on promoting family functioning must not only address the challenges and internalized stigma that affected energy and self-esteem, but should also promote the development of health-seeking behaviors. Otherwise, unhealthy family functioning may result in families with lower level of commitment to themselves, less sense of control in their lives, and less of a tendency to view change as a positive life challenge.

Family support. Family support may be a crucial factor for the family of children with a disability (Bailey, Skinner, Rodrguez, Gut, & Correa, 1999; Haveman, 1997; Sayger & Bowersox, 1996). Support from significant others and social support both formally and informally positively affect family functioning (Bennett & DeLuca, 1996; Bristol, 1987). Olsen et al. (1999) proposed that family support was positively related to family hardiness for both fathers and mothers with disabled children. A large body of evidence suggests that social support is an important factor in mediating stress and enhancing coping in families of children with disabilities, with considerable support networks outside of the family (Dyson, 1997; Hadadian, 1994; Trivette & Dunst, 1992).

While significant, family support contributed to a small percent unit variance explaining of family functioning (see Table 8) after controlling the other independent variables. But the standardized total effect of family support on family functioning was high because family health and family hardiness were mediators to influence family supports indirect effect on family functioning. Dunst, Trivette, and Deal (1988) reported that informal support results in more optimal family functioning, while Haveman et al. (1997) emphasized the influence of formal support for families of children with disabilities. Other researchers have also found that extra-family resources are important for healthy family functioning.

Summary. The most important findings of the Family Stressors, Resources, and Functioning Model were that four variables directly or indirectly affected family functioning: age when diagnosed with DMD, family hardiness, family support, and family health had direct effects on family functioning and the first three variables had indirect effects on family functioning. However, all four variables accounted for 68% of the variance in family functioning. Failla and Jones (1991) reported that family hardiness, functional support, family stressors, and parental age among families of children with developmental disability accounted for 42% of the variance in family functioning.

In reviewing the study data about direct and indirect effects of predictors on family functioning, the path coefficient between family hardiness and family functioning was in a higher range and in the direction predicted. The association between these two variables was strong when the total combined score and the family functioning score were used. This result is similar to a study that found family hardiness was positively associated with family functioning in parents of children with asthma (Donnelly, 1994). Others have argued that family hardiness and family health are related to family functioning in term of the child's health and severity of symptom (Carpiniello, Piras, Pariante, Carta, & Rudas, 1995; Luescher et al., 1999; Walker, Van Slyke, & Newbrough, 1992). The positive relationship between hardiness and healthy family functioning suggests that parents of children with DMD who had greater internal strengths to endure stressors also had greater health. In addition, from a health promotion perspective, the findings support the development of family hardiness through family support services that could be incorporated into health promotion programs in the long-term.

Predictive Variables Effect on Family Health

Family support and family hardiness were predictors, which were direct and indirect effect on family health. One report suggests that families with low family support had significantly higher psychosocial dysfunction than families with adequate family support (Murphy et al., 1998). Family hardiness was found to influence perceived psychological distress; and supportive social resources might directly affect functioning among parents with disabled children (Sloper, 1999), parents with a developmental disability (Failla & Jones, 1991), and family of children with disability (Snowdon et al., 1994). Bigbee (1992) found that hardiness may have a direct effect as well as a buffering effect in the stress-illness relationship. Several authors proposed that hardiness functions as a buffer or mediating factor that may enhance coping or reduce harmful effects of stress (Failla & Jones, 1991; H. I. McCubbin et al., 1996). In addition, family hardiness also has been found to be a significant factor in health promotion (Donnelly, 1994). These findings suggested that health promotion should focus on the creation of interventions to strengthen family hardiness and support.

Predictive Variables Effect on Family Hardiness

Access to care and family support influenced family hardiness (see figure 7). The results of hierarchical multiple regressions showed that earlier diagnosis with DMD was associated with healthier family functioning and better family hardiness. All the total effects of age when diagnosed with DMD and family support on family hardiness were derived from their individual influence of direct effect on family hardiness.

Summary

The study was based on the conceptualization of several factors thought to influence the variables of family stressors (child disability and access to care), family resources (family hardiness, family support, family health, and family characteristics) on the outcome variable family functioning. Results of testing supported the predicted relationships between the age when diagnosed with DMD and family functioning; they also supported the predicted relationships between family hardiness and family functioning, family health and family functioning, and family support and family functioning. The findings support the recommendation that family stress, family resources, and family functioning be operationalized as complex univariates.

Limitations of the study included the non-probability and cross-sectional design. The sample was drawn mostly from TMDA. This sample reflected the middle-aged parents of DMD families at that time. At the time of the study, a great majority of the sample had benefited resources and information from the TMDA. The findings of this study might have been different if the respondent had been drawn from non TMDA families with DMD children, where the level of disability, family annual income, and family hardiness might have differed from the sample. Although duration of illness and length of time in treatment did not correlate, or predict family hardiness, family support, family health, and family functioning, conclusions about time effects are limited by the cross-sectional design of the study.

The majority of the respondents had such similar characteristics that made it difficult to do multivariate analysis for the demographic independent variables, only by dummy coding to dichotomy categories. Thus, the participants may have over reported family support; and underreported family hardiness and family functioning. Limited attention has been given to families with DMD children, although they are a particularly vulnerable population. Other families not participating in TMDA may have different responses.

Sample size was not enough to explore the relationship and do the hierarchical regression among the subscales of each measurement. All these factors limit the generalizability of the findings to other samples of families whose children are reported as disabled. This study needs to be replicated with a longitudinal design that samples both men and women who have a handicapped child. The study did not provide a picture of family functioning from the perspective from all family members. Therefore, it is not known how family functioning or family health would correlate with family hardiness as reported by other family members.

Contribution to Nursing Knowledge

Knowledge of the Resilience Model and the Model of Family Stressors, Resources, and Functioning can be useful in nursing practice. A family centered and strength-based approach is needed with a focus on resources and skills to provide loving and caring relationships, effective communication, and empowerment of the family and community in building resilience. Social networks have an effect on family adaptation. Professionals can explore family support, family communication, and family hardiness in families with children with disabilities to help families develop insights and behaviors associated with hardiness. The Model can be used to evaluate outcomes of interventions that are designed to minimize threats to family integrity and to facilitate healthy adaptation in caring for a child with special needs. These findings further suggest that interventions are needed to improve communication skills, affective expression, and behavior control training.

Clinical Practice Implications

The findings from this investigation provide some important targets for nursing practice with families who have disabled children. From a clinical perspective, this model addresses many of the variables that nurses confront when evaluating family nursing interventions. Clinicians who use the Family Resiliency Model or the Family Stressors, Resources, and Functioning Model could modify their interventions to build on the family's strengths and improve functioning. For example, it would be reasonable to assess parents' health status and focus interventions on clinical services that are convenient and affordable. It would be important to provide training on communication skills, affective expression, and parenting skills to alleviate anxiety and depression, and improve self-esteem and mental-social health. This training should take place over several weeks to allow time for the development of trust and therapeutic relationship.

The culmination of family data yields a family nursing diagnosis that may be focused on the individual parent and how he or she might help meet illness demands, or it may address the family's need for information, resources, problem-solving, education, or role negotiation. The importance of the earlier detection of the disease for faster to access to professional care needs to be emphasized, including prenatal and neonatal screening programs.

Implication for Nursing Education

Nursing educators should foster knowing about DMD, genetic counseling, screening, health promotion, as well as provide students with the opportunity to assess and care for DMD children and their families. With this foundation, students will begin to appreciate the need for family, school, and community interventions that can support DMD children and their families. Findings from this study can enhance curricula related to family strength-based approaches to children with disabilities or chronic illnesses and their families.

Contributions of Family Process Research

A systemic view of hardiness and family functioning is important to understand how individuals, couples, and families cope and adapt through crisis and adversity. The family resilience framework provides theoretical understanding about how family resiliency and family functioning are related. This understanding can usefully inform our efforts to strengthen families in distress. The search for family resiliency and family functioning should identify key processes that can strengthen each family's ability to overcome the challenges they face in their particular life situation. Family resilience-oriented interventions in clinical practice should build on the principles and techniques common among strength-based approaches and should be systematically evaluated. Using psychometrically distinct measures of problem solving, communication, and affective responsiveness would strengthen future studies.

This study used instruments that had been previously used with other populations. The results suggest that the responses of parents of children with DMD fall within the normal range when compared with other populations. An important outcome of this study was the information on the cross-culturally validity of the instruments used. Yet the study also challenges researchers to pursue the development of instruments that are more culturally sensitive and cultural competent. Longitudinal studies have suggested that in some families of children with disabilities, symptoms of distress are chronic and persistent. Further research should begin to focus on specific interventions to improve family functioning, especially in families with later access to care.

REFERENCES

Acreman, M. E. (2002). *Childhood resilience in the academic setting.* Unpublished doctoral dissertation, Queen's University at Kingston (CANADA), Kingston, Ontario.

Adrian, S. (2002). Disability defined. *Psychology Today, 35,* 34.

Alcantara, M. A., Garcia-Cavazos, R., Hernandez, U. E., Gonzalez-del Angel, A., Carnevale, A., & Orozco, L. (2001). Carrier detection and prenatal molecular diagnosis in a Duchenne muscular dystrophy family without any affected relative available. *Annales de Genetique., 44*(3), 149-153.

Antonovsky, A., & Sourani, T. (1988). Family sense of coherence. *Journal of Marriage and the Family, 50,* 79-92.

Appleton, R. E., & Nicolaides, P. (1995). Early diagnosis of Duchenne muscular dystrophy. *Lancet, 345,* 1243-1244.

Baigas, H. R. (2002). *Families and learning in classified and non-classified first graders.* Unpublished doctoral dissertation, Seton Hall University.

Bailey, D. B., Skinner, D., Rodrguez, P., Gut, D., & Correa, V. (1999). Awareness, use, and satisfaction with services for Latino parents of young children with disabilities. *Exceptional children, 65,* 367-381.

Bakker, J. P. J., de Groot, I. J. M., Beelen, A., & Lankhorst, G. J. (2002). Predictive factors of cessation of ambulation in patients with Duchenne muscular dystrophy. *American Journal Physical Medical Rehabilitation, 81,* 906-912.

Beavers, W. R., & Hampson, R. B. (1993). Measuring family competence: The Beavers System Model. In F. Walsh (Ed.), *Normal family processes* (2 ed., pp. 73-95). New York: Guilford.

Bennett, T., & DeLuca, D. A. (1996). Families of children with disabilities: Positive adaptation across the life cycle. *Social Work in Education, 18,* 31- 44.

Beresford, B. (1994). *Positive parents: Caring for a severely disabled child.* London: SRNU, HMSO.

Bernstein, L., Garbin, C., & McClellan, P. (1983). A confirmatory factoring of the California Psychological inventory. *Educational and Psychological Measurement, 43,* 687-691.

Berry, C. (2004). *Family Resiliency: Woman's issues, family travel, and family issues.* Retrieved March, 12, 2004, from the World Wide Web: www.christyberry.org/family_resiliency.htm

Bigbee, J. L. (1992). Family stress, hardiness, and illness: A pilot study. *Family Relations, 41,* 212-217.

Bothwell, J. E., Dooley, J. M., Gordon, K. E., MacAuley, A., Camfield, P. R., & MacSween, J. (2002). Duchenne muscular dystrophy: Parental perceptions. *Clinical Pediatrics, 41*(2), 105-109.

Botvin, M. J. G., Radford, L. M., & Neumann, E. M. (1984). Psychosocial aspects of death and dying in Duchenne muscular dystrophy. *Archieve of Physical Medical Rehabilitation, 65*, 79-82.

Bradley, D. M., Parsons, E. P., & Clarke, A. J. (1993). Experience with screening newborns for Duchenne muscular dystrophy in Wales. *British Medical Journal, 306*, 357-360.

Braverman, M. T. (2001). *Family resiliency: Building strengths to meet life's changes.* Focus: Spring.

Bristol, M. M. (1987). Mothers of children with autism or communication disorders: Successful adaptation and the Double ABCX Model. *Journal of Autism and Developmental Disorders, 17*, 469-486.

Bristor, M. M. (1991). The birth of a handicapped child: A wholistic model for grieving. In A. E. Dell Orto (Ed.), *The psychological and social impact of disability* (pp. 59-80). New York: Springer.

Browne, G. B., Arpin, K., Coey, P., Fitch, M., & Gafni, A. (1990). Prevalence and correlates of family dysfunction and poor adjustment to chronic illness in specially clinics. *Journal of Clinical Epidemiology, 43*, 373-383.

Bubolz, M. M., & Whiren, A. P. (1984). The family of the handicapped: An ecological model for policy and practice. *Family Relations, 33*(5-12).

Buchanan, D., LaBarbera, C., Roelofs, R., & Olson, W. (1979). Reactions of families to children with Duchenne muscular dystrophy. *General Hospital Psychiatry, 3*, 262-269.

Burden, R. (1991). Psycho-social transitions in the lives of parents of children with handicapping conditions. *Counseling Psychology Quarterly, 4*, 331-343.

Byles, J., Bryne, C., Bolye, M., & Offord, D. R. (1988). Ontario child health study: Reliability and validity of the General Functioning subscale of the McMaster Family Assessment Device. *Family Process, 27*, 97-104.

Campbell, C., & Demi, A. (2000). Adult children of fathers missing in action (MIA): An examination of emotional distress, grief, and family hardiness. *Family Relations, 49*, 267-276.

Canning, R. D., Harris, E. S., & Kelleher, K. J. (1996). Factors predicting distress among caregivers to children with chronic health medical conditions. *Journal of Pediatric Psychology, 21*, 735-749.

Cannors, J. L., & Donnellan, A. M. (1998). Walk in beauty: Western perspectives on disability and Navajo family / cultural resilience. In J. E. Fromer (Ed.), *Resiliency in Native America and immigrant families* (pp. 159-182). Thousand Oaks, CA: Sage.

Carey, P. J., Oberst, M. T., McCubbin, A., & Hughes, S. H. (1991). Appraisal and caregiving burden in family members caring for patients receiving chemotherapy. *Oncology Nursing Forum, 18*, 1341-1348.

Carpiniello, B., Piras, A., Pariante, C. M., Carta, M. G., & Rudas, N. (1995). Psychiatric morbidity and family burden among parents of disabled children. *Psychiatric Service, 46*, 940-942.

Chen, J. L. (2002). *Factors associated with children's health in Taiwan and the United States.* Unpublished doctoral dissertation, University of California, San Francisco, San Francisco.

Chen, J. L., & Liu, J. T. (1989). *Family function assessment of psychiatric patients: Second year's study* (RB78-1340). Taipei, Taiwan: STIC, National Science Committee.

Chen, J. Y. (1988). A study of the hospitalized children's stress by projective technique. *Kaohsiung Journal of Medical Sciences, 4*(4), 207-216.

Chen, J. Y., Chen, S. S., Jong, Y. J., & Yang, Y. H. (2002). *The impact for the parents with Ducehnne muscular dystrophy children.*Unpublished manuscript.

Chen, J. Y., Chen, S. S., Jong, Y. J., Yang, Y. H., & Lue, Y. J. (2003, April 10-12). *Psychosocial stress and coping strategies of parents with Duchenne muscular dystrophy children during the middle stage.* Paper presented at the 36th Annual Communicating Nursing Research Conference & 17th Annual Win Assembly, Scottsdale Arizona.

Chen, Y. C., Chen, C. C., Hsu, S. H., & Lin, C. C. (1980). A preliminary study of Family APGAR Index. *Acta Pediatric Sinica, 21*, 210-216.

Cohen, J. (1988). *Statistical power analysis for the behavioral sciences* (2 ed.). Hillsdale, New Jersey: Lawrence Erlbaum Associates.

Cohen, O., Slonim, I., Finzi, R., & Leichtentritt, R. D. (2002). Family resilience: Israeli mothers' perspectives. *American Journal of Family Therapy, 30*, 173-187.

Collin, C., Wade, D. T., Davis, S., & Horne, V. (1988). The Barthel ADL index: A reliability study. *International Disability Studies, 10*, 61-63.

Damrosch, S. P., & Perry, L. A. (1989). Self-reported adjustment, chronic sorrow, and coping of parents of children with Down syndrome. *Nursing Research., 38*(1), 25-30.

Dare, C., & Key, A. (1999). Family functioning and adolescent anorexia nervosa. *British Journal of Psychiatry, 175*(7), 89.

Department of Health, Taiwan R. O. C. (2001). *Crude birth rates, crude death rates and natural increase rates, Taiwan area, 1962-2001.* Health and national health insurance annual statistics information service. Retrieved January 23, 2003, from the World Wide Web: http://www.doh.gov.tw/statistic/data

Donnelly, E. (1994). Parents of children with asthma: An examination of family hardiness, family stressors, and family functioning. *Journal of Pediatric Nursing, 9*(6), 398-408.

Dunst, C. J., Trivete, C. M., & Deal, A. G. (1988). *Enabling and empowering families: Principles and guidelines for practice.* Cambridhe, MA: Brookline Books.

Dyson, L. L. (1997). Fathers and mothers of school-age children with developmental disabilities: Parental stress, family functioning and social support. *American Journal on Mental Retardation, 102,* 267-279.

Emery, A. E. H. (1993). *Duchenne muscular dystrophy* (2 ed.). Oxford: Oxford Medical Publish.

Emery, A. E. H. (2002). The muscular dystrophies. *Lancet, 359*(9307), 687.

Epstein, N. B., Baldwin, L. M., & Bishop, D. S. (1983). The McMaster Family Assessment Device. *Journal of Marital and Family Therapy, 9,* 171-180.

Epstein, N. B., Bishop, D. S., & Levin, S. (1978). The McMaster Model of Family Functioning. *Journal of Marriage and Family Counseling, 4,* 19-31.

Epstein, N. B., Bishop, D. S., Ryan, C. E., Miller, I. W., & Keitner, G. I. (1993). The McMaster Model: View of healthy family functioning. In F. Walsh (Ed.), *Normal family processes* (pp. 138-160). New York: Guilford.

Epstein, N. B., Bishop, D. S., Ryan, C. E., Miller, I. W., & Keitner, G. I. (2003). The McMaster Model: View of healthy family functioning. In F. Walsh (Ed.), *Normal family processes* (pp. 581-607). New York: Guilford.

Failla, S., & Jones, L. C. (1991). Families of children with developmental disabilities: An examination of family hardiness. *Research in Nursing and Health, 14,* 41-50.

Firth, M. A., Gardner-Medwin, D., Hosking, G., & Wilkinson, E. (1983). Interviews with parents of boys suffering from Duchenne muscular dystrophy. *Development Medicine and Child Neurology, 25,* 466-471.

Fitzpatrick, C., & Barry, C. (1986). Psychiatric disorder among boys with Duchenne muscular dystrophy. *Developmental Medicine and Child Neurology, 28,* 589-595.

Fitzpatrick, C., & Barry, C. (1990). Cultural differences in family communication about Duchenne muscular dystrophy. *Developmental Medicine and Child Neurology, 32*, 967-973.

Fornari, V., Wlodarczyk-Bisaga, K., Matthews, M., Sandberg, D. M., F. S., & Katz, J. L. (1999). Perception of family functioning and depressive symptomatology in individuals with anorexia nervosa or bulimia nervosa. *Comprehensive Psychiatry, 40*, 434-441.

Foulke, F. G., Reeb, K. G., Graham, A. V., & Zyzanski, S. J. (1988). Family function, respiratory illness, and otitis media in urban black infants. *Family Medicine., 20*(2), 128-132.

Freedman, M. (1979). The politics of an old state: A view from the Chinese lineage. In G. W. Skinner (Ed.), *The study of Chinese society: Essays by Maurice Freedman*. Stanford: Stanford University.

Friedmann, M. S., McDermut, W. H., Solomon, D. A., Ryan, C. E., Keitner, G. I., & Miller, I. W. (1997). Family functioning and mental illness: A comparison of psychiatric and nonclinical families. *Family Process, 36*, 357-367.

Gagliardi, B. A. (1991). The family's experience of living with a child with Duchenne muscular dystrophy. *Applied Nursing Research, 4*(4), 159-164.

Gardner, W., Nutting, P. A., Kelleher, K. J., Werner, J. J., Farley, T., Stewart, L., Hartsell, M., & Orzano, A. J. (2001). Does the family APGAR effectively measure family functioning? *Journal of Family Practice, 50*(1), 19-25.

Garwick, A. W., Kohrman, C. H., Titus, J. C., Wolman, C., & Blum, R. W. (1999). Variations in families' explanations of childhood chronic conditions: A cross cultural perspective. In J. A. Futrell (Ed.), *The dynamics of resilient families* (pp. 165-202). Thousand Oaks, CA: Sage.

Gillis, C. L., Neuhaus, J. M., & Hauck, W. W. (1990). Improving family functioning after cardiac surgery: A randomized trial. *Heart & Lung: Journal of Acute & Critical Care, 19*(6), 648-654.

Glantz, S. A., & Slinker, B. K. (1990). *Primer of applied regression and analysis of variance*. New York: McGraw-Hill.

Gold, T. B. (1996). Taiwan society at the Fin de Siecle. In D. Shambaugh (Ed.), *Contemporary Taiwan* (pp. 47-70). Oxford: Clarendon.

Good, M. D., Smilkstein, G., Good, B. J., Shaffer, T., & Arons, T. (1979). The Family APGAR Index: A study of construct validity. *Journal of Family Practice, 8*(3), 577-582.

Gottlieb, A. (1998). Single mother of children with disabilities: The role of sense of coherence in managing multiple challenges. In J. E. Fromer (Ed.), *Stress, coping, and health in families: Sense of coherence and resiliency* (pp. 189-206). Thousand Oak, California: Sage.

Gowers, S., & North, C. (1999). Difficulties in family functioning and adolescent anorexia nervosa. *British Journal of Psychiatry, 174*(1), 63-66.

Gragert, M., & Ide, B. A. (2003). *Reliability and validity of a revised family disruption from Illness scale in a rural sample.* Online Journal of Rural Nursing and Health Care. Retrieved January, 2, 2004, from the World Wide Web: http://www.rno.org/journal/volume2/issue2/ide.html

Greenhalgh, S. (1984). Networks and their nodes: Urban society on Taiwan. *The China Quartely, 99*, 529-552.

Gwyther, R. E., Bentz, E. J., Drossman, D. A., & Berolzheimer, N. (1993). Validity of the Family APGAR in patients with irritable bowel syndrome. *Family Medicine., 25*(1), 21-25.

Hadadian, A. (1994). Stress and social support in fathers and mothers of young children with and without disabilities. *Early Education and Development, 5*, 226-235.

Hair, J. F., Anderson, R. E., Tatham, R. L., & Black, W. C. (1998). *Multivariate data analysis.* Upper Saddle River, New Jersey: Prentice Hall.

Haveman, M. (1997). Difference inservice needs, time demand, and caregiving burden among parents with mental retardation across the life cycle. *Family Relation, 46*, 417- 425.

Hawley, D. R. (2000). Clinical implications of family resilience. *American Journal of Family Therapy, 28*, 101-126.

Hayden, L. C., Schiller, M., Dickstein, S., Seifer, R., Sameroff, A. J., Rhode, I. M., Keitner, G., & Rasmussen, S. (1998). Levels of family assessment: I. Family, marital, and parent-child interaction. *Journal of Family Psychology, 12*(1), 7-22.

Henkle, E. J. (1994). *Hardiness, burden, stress, appraisal, coping and well-being of family caregivers of homebound older adults.* Unpublished Doctoral Dissertation, Indiana University, Indiana.

Heru, A. M., & Ryan, C. E. (2002). Depressive symptoms and family functioning in the caregivers of recently hospitalized patients with chronic/recurrent mood disorders. *International Journal of Psychosocial Rehabilitation, 7,* 53-60.

Hilliard, R., Gjerde, C., & Parker, L. (1986). Validity of two psychological screening measures in family practice: Personal Inventory and Family APGAR. *Journal of Family Practice, 23*(4), 345-349.

Hoffman, E. P., Brown, R. H. J., & Kunkel, L. M. (1987). Dystrophin: The protein product of the Duchenne muscular dystrophy locus. *Cell, 51,* 919-928.

Holroyd, J., & Guthrie, D. (1979). Stress in families of children with neuromuscular disease. *Journal of Clinical Psychology, 35*(4), 734-739.

Huang, C. F. (1996). *Families of children with developmental disabilities: The test of a structural model of family hardiness, social support, stress, coping, and family functioning.* Unpublished doctoral dissertation, Saint Louis University, Saint Louis.

Huang, D. X. (1994). *Family dysfunctioning with role maladjustment and drug abuse in adolescence.* Unpublished master's thesis, Soochow University, Taipei, Taiwan.

Huang, L., & Dai, Y. (1998). Psychosocial impact of muscular dystrophy on mothers [Chinese]. *Journal of Nursing Research (China), 6*(2), 137-151.

Institute for Health and Disability. (1997). A new way to think about cultural sensitivity: Families share their understanding of disabilities. *Health Issues for Children & Youth and Their Family, 5*(1), 1-12.

Jakubiczka, S., Mitulla, B., Liehr, T., Arnemann, J., Lehrach, H., Sudbrak, R., Stumm, M., Wieacker, P. F., & Bettecken, T. (2000). Incidental prenatal detection of an Xp deletion using an anonymous primer pair for fetal sexing. *Prenatal Diagnosis., 20*(10), 842-846.

Judge, S. L. (1998). Parental coping strategies and strengths in families of young childen with disabilities. *Family Relations, 47,* 262-267.

Kabacoff, R. I., Miller, I. W., Bishop, D. S., Epstein, N. B., & Keitner, G. I. (1990). A psychometric study of the McMaster family assessment device in psychiatric, medical, and nonclinical samples. *Journal of Family Psychology, 3,* 431-439.

Kamya, H. A. (1997). African immigrants in the United States: The challenge for research and practice. *Social Work, 42*(2), 154-165.

Kao, P. L. (1998). *Social support, caregiving burden and quality of life of the parents with Duchenne Muscular Dystrophy Children.* Unpublished Master's Thesis, Kaohsiung Medial University, Kaohsiung, Taiwan.

Keitner, G. I. (1990). *Depression and families: Impact and treatment*. Washington: American Psychiatric.

Keitner, G. I., Fodor, J., Ryan, C. E., Miller, I. W., Epstein, N. B., & Bishop, D. S. (1991). A cross-cultural study of major depression and family functioning. *Canadian Journal of Psychiatry, 36*, 254-258.

Keitner, G. I., Miller, I. W., & Ryan, C. E. (1993). The role of the family in major depressive illness. *Psychiatric Annals, 23*(9), 500-507.

Keitner, G. I., Ryan, C. E., Miller, I. W., Kohn, R., Bishop, D. S., & Epstein, N. B. (1995). Role of the family in recovery and major depression. *American Journal of Psychiatry, 152*(7), 1002-1008.

Keitner, G. I., Ryan, C. E., Miller, I. W., & Norman, W. H. (1992). Recovery and major depression. *American Journal of Psychiatry, 149*(1), 93-98.

Kenneth, M. (2001). Disability. *Journal of Medical Ethics, 27*(6), 361-362.

Khamis, V. (1998). Psychological distress and well-being among traumatized palestinian women during the intifada. *Social Science Medicine, 46*(8), 1033-1041.

Kilmer, D. D., Abresch, R. T., & Fowler, W. M. J. (1993). Serial manual muscle testing in Duchenne muscular dystrophy. *Archieve Physical Medicine Rehabilitation, 74*, 1168-1171.

Kim, H. Y. (2002). *The relationship of stressors and family resources to family functioning.* Unpublished doctoral dissertation, University of Alberta, Canada.

King, C. A., Segal, H. G., Naylor, M., & Evans, T. (1993). Family functioning and suicidal behavior in adolescent inpatients with mood disorders. *Journal of the American Academy of Child & Adolescent Psychiatry, 32*(6), 1198-1206.

Kirkevold, M., Gortner, S. R., Berg, K., & Saltvold, S. (1996). Patterns of recovery among Norwegian heart surgery patients. *Journal of Advanced Nursing, 24*, 943-951.

Knussen, C., & Sloper, P. (1992). Stress in families of children with disability: A review of risk and resistance factors. *Journal of Mental Health, 1*, 241-256.

Kobasa, S. C. (1979). Stressful life events, personality, and health: An Inquiry into hardiness. *Journal of Personality and Social Psychology, 37*, 1-11.

Kosciulek, J. F., McCubbin, M. A., & McCubbin, H. I. (1993). A theoretical framework for family adaptation to head injury. *Journal of Rehabilitation, 59*, 40-45.

Kuo, S. C. (2000). *The contribution of the preterm labor stress and family resiliency factors to pregnancy adjustment and adaptation in the preterm labor family.* Unpublished Doctoral Dissertation, University of Wisconsin, Madison, Wisconsin.

Ladewig, B. H., & Jessee, P. O. (1992). Children held hostage: Mothers' depressive affect and perceptions of family psychosocial. *Journal of Family Issues, 13*, 65-71.

Laing, N. G. (1993). Molecular genetics and genetic counseling for Duchenne /Becker muscular dystrophy. In T. Patridge (Ed.), *Molecular and cell biology of muscular dystrophy* (pp. 37-84). London: Chapman & Hall.

Lambert, C. E. J., & Lambert, V. A. (1999). Psychological hardiness: State of the science. *Holistic Nursing Practice, 13*, 11-19.

Lambert, V. A., Lambert, C. E., Klipple, G. L., & Mewshaw, E. A. (1990). Relationships among hardiness, social support, severity of illness, and psychological well being in women with rheumatoid arthritis. *Health Care Women International, 11*, 159-173.

Lampher, B. E. (1999). *Perception of family functioning as it relates to suicidal thoughts and behavior of adolescents.* Unpublished Doctoral Dissertation, University of Akron, Arkon, Ohio.

Lee, M. B. (1991). *A medical-psychiatric liaison program for cardiac inpatients: Establishment of model and evaluation* (RC8410-1013). Taipei, Taiwan: STIC, National Science Committee.

Lee, M. B. (1999). *Psychosomatic study on HIV-1 infected patients: The seventh year* (RG9010-0119). Taipei, Taiwan: STIC, National Science Committee.

Lee, M. B., Chuang, C. Y., & Shen, M. C. (1994). *Psychosomatic study on HIV-1 infected patients (III)* (RB8504-1215). Taipei, Taiwan: STIC, National Science Committee.

Lee, M. B., & Lin, S. (1989). *Prospective follow-up study of neurosis: Course, outcome, and prognostic factors.* (RC77-5065). Taipei, Taiwan: STIC, National Science Committee.

Leske, J. S. (2000). Family stresses, strengths, and outcomes after critical injury. *Critical Care Nursing Clinics of North America, 12*(2), 237-244.

Leske, J. S. (2003). Comparison of family stresses, strengths, and outcomes after trauma and surgery. *AACN Clinical Issues: Advanced Practice in Acute & Critical Care, 14*(1), 33-41.

Leske, J. S., & Jiricka, M. K. (1998). Impact of family demands and family strengths and capabilities on family well-being and adaptation after critical injury. *American Journal of Critical Care, 7*(5), 383-392.

Lieb, R., Wittchen, H.-U., Hofler, M. D., Fuetsch, M. M., Stein, M. B., & Merikangas, K. R. (2000). Parental psychopathology, parenting styles, and the risk of social phobia in offspring: A prospective-longitudinal community study. *Archives of General Psychiatry, 57*(9), 859-866.

Lin, M. (1990). Greater demand for size XL. *Free China Review, 40,* 49-51.

Lindeman, S., Kaprio, J., Isometsa, K., Poikolainen, M., Heikkinen, M., Hamalainen, J., Haarasilta, T., Laukkala, T., & Aro, H. (2002). Spousal Resemblance for history of major depressive episode in the previous year. *Psychological Medicine, 32,* 363-367.

Loder, R. T., Warschausky, S., Schwartz, E. M., Hensinger, R. N., & Greenfield, M. L. (1995). The psychosocial characteristics of children with fractures. *Journal of Pediatric Orthopedics, 15*(1), 41-46.

Long-Term Care Profession Association of ROC. (1997). *The list of registered long-term care services in Taiwan.* Taipei, Taiwan. (in Chinese): Long-term Care Profession Association of ROC.

Lue, Y. J., Chen, S. S., Jong, Y. J., & Lin, Y. T. (1993). Investigation of activity of daily living performance in patients with Duchenne Muscular Dystrophy. *Kaohsiung Journal Medical Science, 9,* 351-360.

Luescher, J. L., Dede, D. E., Gitten, J. C., Fennell, E., & Maria, B. L. (1999). Parental burden, coping, and family functioning in primary caregivers of children with Joubert syndrome. *Journal of Child Neurology, 14,* 642-648.

Lustig, D. (1997). Families with an adult with mental retardation: Empirical family typologies. *Rehabilitation Counseling Bulletin, 41,* 138-157.

Magill-Evans, J., Darrah, J., Pain, K., Adkins, R., & Kratochvil, M. (2001). Are families with adolescents and young adults with cerebral palsy the same as other families? *Developmental Medicine & Child Neurology, 43,* 466-472.

Mahoney, F. I., & Barthel, D. W. (1965). Functional evaluation: the Barthel Index. *Maryland State Medical Journal, 14,* 56-61.

Margalit, M., Raviv, A., & Ankonina, D. B. (1992). Coping and coherence among parents with disabled children. *Journal of Clinical Child Psychology, 21,* 202-209.

Marsh, R. M. (1996). *Taiwan in the modern world: The great transformation: Social change in Taipei, Taiwan since the 1960s.* Armonk, New York: M. E. Sharpe.

Martin, G., Rozanes, P., Pearce, C., & Allison, S. (1995). Adolescent suicide, depression and family dysfunctioning. *Acta Psychiatrica Scandinavia, 92,* 336-344.

Max, J. E., Castillo, C. S., Robin, D. A., Lindgren, S. D., Smith, W. L. J., Sato, Y., Mattheis, P. J., & Stierwalt, J. A. G. (1998). Predictors of family functioning after traumatic brain injury in children and adolescents. *Journal of the American Academy of Child & Adolescent Psychiatry, 37*(1), 83-90.

McCallion, P., & Toseland, R. W. (1993). Empowering families of adolescents and adults with developmental disabilities. *Families in Society, 74*, 579-587.

McCubbin, H. I. (1998). Resiliency in African American families: Military families in foreign environments. In J. A. Futrell (Ed.), *Resiliency in African-American families.* Thousand Oaks, CA: Sage.

McCubbin, H. I., & McCubbin, M. A. (1988). Typologies of resilient families: Emerging roles of social class and ethnicity. *Family Relations, 37*, 247-254.

McCubbin, H. I., McCubbin, M. A., Thompson, A. I., Han, S. Y., & Allen, C. T. (1997, June 22). *Families under stress: What makes them resilient.* Paper presented at the 1997 American Association of Family and Consumer Sciences Commemorative Lecture, Washington, D. C.

McCubbin, H. I., McCubbin, M. A., Thompson, A. I., & Thompson, E. I. (1998). Resiliency in ethic families: A conceptual model for predicting family adjustment and adaptation. In J. E. Fromer (Ed.), *Resiliency in native American and immigrant families* (pp. 3-48). Thousands Oaks, CA: Sage.

McCubbin, H. I., & Thompson, A. I. (1991). *Family assessment inventories for reseach and practice.* Madison: University of Wisconsin.

McCubbin, H. I., Thompson, A. I., & McCubbin, M. A. (1996). *Family assessment: Resiliency, coping, and adaptation: Inventories for research and practice.* Madison, WI: University of Wisconsin System.

McCubbin, H. I., Thompson, A. I., & McCubbin, M. A. (2001). *Family measures: Stress, coping, and resiliency --Inventories for research and practice.* Honolulu, Hawaii: Kamehameha Schools.

McCubbin, H. I., Thompson, A. I., Thompson, E. A., Elver, K. M., & McCubbin, M. A. (1998). Ethnicity, schema, and coherence: Appraisal processes for families in crisis. In J. E. Fromer (Ed.), *Stress, coping, and health in families: Sense of coherence and resiliency* (pp. 41-67). Madison, Wisconsin: University of Wisconsin.

McCubbin, M. A., & McCubbin, H. I. (1991). Family stress theory and assessment: The resiliency model of family stress, adjustment, and adpatation. In A. I. Thompson (Ed.), *Family assessment inventories for research and practice* (pp. 3-34). Madison: University of Wisconsin.

McCubbin, M. A., & McCubbin, H. I. (1993). Families coping with illness: The resiliency model of family stress, adjustment, and adaptation. In P. Winstead-Fry (Ed.), *Families, health, & illness: Perspectives on coping and intervention* (pp. 21-63). St. Louis: Mosby.

McCubbin, M. A., McCubbin, H. I., & Thompson, A. I. (1986). Family Hardiness Index (FHI). In M. A. McCubbin (Ed.), *Family assessment: Resiliency, coping and adaptation-Inventories for research and practice* (pp. 239-306). Madison: University of Wisconsin System.

McCubbin, M. A., McCubbin, H. I., & Thompson, A. I. (1996). Family problem solving communication (FPSC). In M. A. McCubbin (Ed.), *Family assessment: Resiliency, coping, and adaptation: Inventories for research and practice* (pp. 639-686). Madison: University of Wisconsin.

McFarlane, A. H., Bellissimo, A., & Norman, G. R. (1995). Family structure, family functioning and adolescent well-being: The transcendent influence of parental style. *Journal of Child Psychology and Psychiatry, 36*, 847-864.

McGoldrick, M., & Carter, B. (2003). The family life cycle. In F. Walsh (Ed.), *Normal family process* (3 ed., pp. 375-398). New York: Guilford.

McIntyre, C. L. (2000). *The role of competency-enhancing helpgiving practice in parental adaptation for families of children with special needs.* Unpublished Doctoral Dissertation, University of Texas at Austin, Austin, Texas.

Medical Outcome Trust. (2001). *Freuently asked uestions about the Duke.* Retrieved February 28, 2003, from the World Wide Web: http://www.outcomes-trust.org/instruments/DUKEfreq.htm

Mellon, S., & Northouse, L. L. (2001). Family survivorship and quality of life following a cancer diagnosis. *Research in Nursing & Health, 24*, 446-459.

Merikangas, K. R., Avenevoli, S., Dierker, L., & Grillon, C. (1999). Vulnerability factors among children at risk for anxiety disorders. *Biological Psychiatry, 46*, 1523-1535.

Miller, I. V., Epstein, N. B., Bishop, D. S., & Keitner, G. I. (1985). The McMaster Family Assessment Device: Reliability and validity. *Journal of Marital and Family Therapy, 11*, 345-356.

Miller, I. W., Keitner, G. I., Whisman, M. A., Ryan, C. E., Epstein, N. B., & Bishop, D. S. (1992). Depressed patients with dysfunctional families: Description and course of illness. *Journal of Abnormal Psychology, 101*(4), 637-646.

Moos, R. H., & Moos, B. S. (1981). *Family Environment Scale Manual.* Palo Alto, CA: Consulting Psychologists.

Murphy, J. M., Kelleher, K., Pagon, R. A., Stulp, C., Nutting, P. A., Jellinek, M. S., Gardner, W., & Child, G. E. (1998). The Family APGAR and psychosocial problems in children: A report from ASPN and PROS. *Journal of Family Practice, 46*(1), 54-64.

Nereo, N. E., Fee, R. J., & Hinton, V. J. (2003). Parental stress in mothers of boys with Ducehnne muscular dystrophy. *Journal of Pediatric Psychology, 28*, 473-484.

Nereo, N. E., & Hinton, V. J. (2003). Three wishes and psychological functioning in boys with Duchenne muscular dystrophy. *Developmental and Behavioral Pediatrics, 24*(2), 96-103.

Newby, N. M. (1996). *Reliability and validity testing of the Family Sense of Coherence Scale in chronic illness.* Unpublished Doctoral Dissertation, Saint Louis University.

Nicholson, L. V. B. (1993). Advances in Duchenne and myotonic dystrophy. *Current Opinion in Rheumatology, 5*, 706-711.

Norris, A. E. (2001). Path analysis. In B. H. Munro (Ed.), *Statistical methods for health care research* (4th ed., pp. 355-377). Philadelphia: Lippincott.

Northouse, L. L., Mood, D., Schafenacker, A., Mellon, S., Walker, J., Galvin, E., & Decker, V. (2002). Quality of life of women with recurrent breast cancer and their family members. *Journal of clinical oncology, 20*, 4050-4064.

O'Farrell, P., Murray, J., & Hotz, S. B. (2000). Psychologic distress among spouses of patients undergoing cardiac rehabilitation. *Heart & Lung: Journal of Acute & Critical Care, 29*(2), 97-104.

Olsen, S. F., Marshall, E. S., Mandleco, B. L., Allred, K. W., Dyches, T. T., & Sansom, N. (1999). Support, communication, and hardiness in families with children with disabilities. *Journal of Family Nursing, 8*, 275-291.

Olson, D., Sprenkle, D., & Russell, C. (1979). Circumplex model of marital and family systems: I. Cohesion and adaptability dimensions, family types and clinical applications. *Family Process, 18*, 3-28.

Olson, D. H. (1993). Circumplex model of marital and family systems: Assessing family functioning. In F. Walsh (Ed.), *Normal family processes* (pp. 104-137). New York: Guildford.

Olson, D. H., Potner, J., & Bell, R. (1982). FACES II: Family Adaptability and Cohesion Evaluation Scales. *St. Paul, MN, Family Social Science, University of Minnesota.*

Pain, H. (1999). Coping with a child with disabilities from the parents' perspective: The function of information. *Child: Care, Health, and Development, 25*, 299-312.

Pal, D. K., Chaudhury, G., Das, T., & Sengupta, S. (2002). Predictors of parental adjustment to children's epilepsy in rural India. *Child: Care, Health & Development, 28,* 295-300.

Palfrey, J. S., Walker, D. K., Butler, J. A., & Singer, J. D. (1989). Patterns of response in families of chronically disabled children: An assessment in five metropolitan school districts. *American Journal of Orthopsychiatric, 59*(1), 94-104.

Parent Project Muscular Dystrophy. (2002). *The basics of muscular dystrophy and beyond: Progression of Duchenne MD.* Retrieved December 12, 2003, from the World Wide Web: www.parentprojectmd.org/aboutdmd/basics/progress.html

Parkerson, G. R. J. (Ed.). (2002). *User's guide for Duke health measures.* Durham, North Carolina: Department of Community and Family Medicine, Duke University Medical Center.

Parkerson, G. R. J., Broadhead, W. E., & Tse, C. K. J. (1991). Comparison of the Duke Health Profile and the MOS Short-form in healthy young adults. *Medical Care, 29,* 679-683.

Patterson, J. M. (2002). *Promoting resilience in families experiencing stress.* University of Minnesota, School of Public Health. Retrieved August 6, 2002, from the World Wide Web: http://www..epi.umi.edu/epi_pages/Syllabi/reading2.html

Patterson, J. M., & McCubbin, H. I. (1983). Chronic illness: Family stress and coping. In H. I. McCubbin (Ed.), *Stress and the family: Volume II: Coping with catastrophe* (pp. 21-36). New York: Brunner/Mazel.

Polit, D. F., & Hunger, B. P. (1999). *Nursing research: Principles and methods.* Philadelphia: J. B. Lippincott.

Ptacek, J. T., Smith, R. E., & Zanas, J. (1992). Gender, appraisal, and coping: A longitudinal analysis. *Journal of Personality, 60,* 747-770.

Reid, D. T., & Renwick, R. M. (2001). Relating familial stress to the psychosocial adjustment of adolescents with Duchenne muscular dystrophy. *International Journal of Rehabilitation Research, 24*(2), 83-93.

Rideau, Y., Duport, G., Delaubier, A., Guillon, C., Renardel-Irani, A., & Bach, J. R. (1995). Early treatment to preserve quality of locomotion for children with Duchenne muscular dystrophy. *Seminar in Neurology, 15,* 9-17.

Rivara, J. M., Jaffe, K. M., Polissar, N. L., Fay, G. C., Liao, S., & Martin, K. M. (1996). Predictors of family functioning and change 3 years after traumatic brain injury in children. *Archives of Physical Medicine & Rehabilitation, 77*(8), 754-764.

Roland, E. H. (2000). Muscular dystrophy. *Pediatric in Review, 21*(7), 233.

Roncone, R., Rossi, L., Muiere, E., Impallomeni, M., Matteucci, M., Giacomelli, R., Tonietti, G., & Casacchia, M. (1998). The Italian version of the Family Assessment Device. *Social Psychiatry and Psychiatric Epidemiology, 33*, 451-461.

Rubin, A., & Babbie, F. (1997). *Research methods for social work*. Grove, CA: Brooks Cole.

Sabbeth, B. (1984). Understanding the impact of chronic childhood illness on families. *Pediatric Clinics of North American, 31*(1), 47-57.

Sawin, J. K., & Harrigan, M. (1994). Measures of family functioning for research and practice. *Scholarly Inquiry for Nursing Practice: An International Journal, 8*(1), 5-142.

Sawin, K. J., & Harrigan, M. P. (1995). *Measures of family functioning for research and practice*. New York: Springer.

Sawyer, M., Sarris, A., Baghurst, P., Cross, D., & Kalucy, R. (1988). Family Assessment Device: Reports from mothers, fathers, and adolescents in community and clinic families. *Journal of Marital and Family Therapy, 14*, 287-296.

Sayger, T. V., & Bowersox, M. P. (1996). Family therapy and the treatment of chronic illness in a multidisciplinary world. *Family Journal, 4*, 12-19.

Scahill, L., Schwab-Stone, M., Merikangas, K. R., Leckman, J. F., Zhang, H., & Kasl, S. (1999). Psychosocial and clinical correlates of ADHD in a community sample of school-age children. *Journal of the American Academy of Child & Adolescent Psychiatry, 38*(8), 976-984.

Schwab, J. J., Gray-Ice, H. M., & Prentice, F. R. (2000). *Family functioning: The general living systems research model*. New York: Kluwer Academic/Plenum.

Seligman, M., & Darling, R. B. (1989). *Ordinary families, special children: A systems approach to childhood disability*. New York: Guilford.

Shah, S., Vanclay, F., & Cooper, B. (1989). Improving the sensitivity of the Barthel Index of stroke rehabilitation. *Journal Clinical Epidemiology, 42*(8), 703-709.

Shek, D. T. L. (2002). Assessment of family functioning in Chinese version of the Family Assessment Device. *Research on Social Work Practice, 12*(4), 502-524.

Shek, D. T. L., Lai, K., & Lai, A. (1998). Assessment of family functioning in Hong Kong. *Hong Kong Journal of Social Work, 32*, 197-199.

Sherwood, S., Morris, J., Mor, V., & et al. (1977). *Compendium of measures for describing and assessing long-term care populations*. Boston: Hebrew Rehabilitation Center for the Aged.

Siciliano, G., Tessa, A., Renna, M., Manca, M. L., Mancuso, M., & Murri, L. (1999). Epidemiology of dystrophinopathies in North-West Tuscany: A molecular genetics-based revisitation. *Clinical Genetics, 56*, 51-58.

Siegel, I. M., Davidson, H., Kornfeld, M., & McCready, W. C. (1983). Coping with muscular dystrophy: Psychosocial correlates of adaptation. *Muscle and Nerve, 6*, 607-609.

Silberberg, S. (2001). Searching for family resilience. *Family Matters, 58*, 52-61.

Silver, C. B. (1982). *Fredric LePlay: On family, work, and social change*. Chicago: University of Chicago.

Sloper, P. (1999). Models of service support for parents of disabled children. What do we know? What do we need to know? *Child: Care, Health, and Development, 25*(2), 85-99.

Smilkstein, G. (1978). The Family APGAR: A proposal for a family function test and its use by physicians. *Journal of Family Practice, 6*(6), 1231-1239.

Smilkstein, G., Ashworth, C., & Montano, D. (1982). Validity and reliability of the Family APGAR as a test of family function. *Journal of Family Practice, 15*, 303-311.

Smith, R. A., Williams, D. K., Sibert, J. R., & Harper, P. S. (1990). Attitude of mothers to neonatal screening for DMD. *British Medicine Journal, 28*, 300.

Smith, S. (1995). Family theory and multicultural family studies. In S. Smith (Ed.), *Families in multicultural perspective* (pp. 5-35). New York: Guilford.

Smith, T. B., & Oliver, M. N. (2001). Parenting stress in families of children with disabilities. *American journal of Orthopsychiatry, 71*, 257-261.

Smucker, W. D., Wildman, B. G., Lynch, T. R., & Revolinsky, M. C. (1995). Relationship between the family AGPAR and behavioral problems in children. *Archieve Family Medicine, 4*, 535-539.

Snowdon, A. W., Cameron, S., & Dunham, K. (1994). Relationships between stress, coping resources, and satisfaction with family functioning in families of children with disabilities. *Canadian Journal of Nursing Research, 26*(3), 63-76.

Stein, D., Williamson, D., Birmaher, B., Brent, D. A., Kaufman, J., Dahl, R. E., Perel, J. M., & Ryan, N. D. (2000). Parent-child bonding and family functioning in depressed children and children at high risk and low risk for future depression. *Journal of the American Academy of Child & Adolescent Psychiatry, 39*, 1387-1395.

Stevenson-Hinde, J., & Akister, J. (1995). The McMaster Model of Family Functioning: Observer and parental ratings in a nonclinical sample. *Family Process, 34*, 337-347.

Summers, J. A., Behr, S. K., & Turnbull, A. P. (1989). Positive adaptation and coping strengths of families: Who have children with disabilities. In L. K. Irvin (Ed.), *Support for caregiving families: Enabling positive adaptation to disability*. Baltimore, MD: Paul H. Brookes.

Suttiamnuaykul, W. (2001). *Measuring family functioning in Thailand: Developing the Thai Family Functioning (TFFS) and comparing psychometric properties to those of the Thai Version of the Family Assessment Device (FAD)*. Unpublished Doctoral Dissertation, University at Buffalo: The State University of New York, New York.

Svavarsdottir, E. K. (1997). *Family adaptation for families of an infant of a young child with asthma*. Unpublished Doctoral Dissertation, University of Wisconsin-Madison, Madison, Wisconsin.

Tamplin, A., & Goodyer, I. M. (2001). Family functioning in adolescents at high and low risk for major depressive disorder. *European Child & Adolescent Psychiatry, 10*, 170-179.

Tamplin, A., Goodyer, I. M., & Herbert, J. (1998). Family functioning and parent general health in families of adolescents with major depressive disorder. *Journal of Affective Disorders, 48*, 1-13.

Tebbutt, J., Swanston, H., Oates, R. K., & O'Toole, B. I. (1997). Five years after child sexual abuse: Persisting dysfunction and problems of prediction. *Journal of the American Academy of Child & Adolescent Psychiatry, 36*(3), 330-339.

Thames, B., & Thomason, D. J. (2000). *Building family strengths resiliency. Clemson Extension: Family Relationships*. Retrieved August, 8, 2002, from the World Wide Web: http://virtual.clemson.edu/groups/psapublishing/Pages/FYD/FL529.pdf

Thompson, R. J. J., Zeman, J. L., Fanurik, D., & Sirotkin-Roses, M. (1992). The role of parent stress and coping and family functioning in parent and child adjustment to Duchenne muscular dystrophy. *Journal of Clinical Psychology, 48*, 11-19.

Thorndike, R. (1978). *Correlational procedures for research*. New York: Gardner Press.

TMDA. (2002). *TMDA bulletin: 019*. Taiwan Muscular Dystrophy Assocition. Retrieved January 23, 2003, from the World Wide Web: tmda.adsldns.org

Traditional Chinese Culture in Taiwan: Philosophy (2002). Retrieved September 21, 2002, from the World Wide Web: http://www.housetoncul.org/culdir/phil/phil.htm

Trivette, C. M., & Dunst, C. J. (1992). Characteristics and influences of role division and social support among mothers of preschool children with disabilities. *Topics in Early Childhood Special Education, 12*, 367-385.

Tsai, M. C., Chang, C. J., & Tseng, W. H. (1993). A preliminary study of reliability and validity of Chinese Version of the Duke Health Profile. *Taiwan Journal of Public Health, 20*(3), 284-295.

Tutty, L. M. (1995). Theoretical and practical issues in selecting a measure of family functioning. *Research on Social Work Practice, 5*, 80-106.

Tyan, M., Chie, W. C., & Chang, C. J. (1988). Illness-Related stress and family support of diabetic patients in Kung-Liao community a preliminary report. *Chinese Journal of Family Medicine, 8*(3), 150-160.

Van der Putten, J. J. M. F., Hobart, J. C., Freeman, J. A., & Thompson, A. J. (1999). Measuring change in disability after inpatient rehabilitation: Comparison of the responsiveness of the Barthel Index and the Functional Independence Measure. *Journal Neurology Neurosurgery Psychiatry, 66*, 480-484.

Vandsburger, E. H. (2001). *The effects of family resiliency resources on the functioning of families experiencing economic distress.* Unpublished doctoral dissertation, Virginia Commonwealth University, Richmond, VA.

Vignos, P. J. J., Wagner, M. B., Karlinchak, B., & Katirji, B. (1996). Evaluation of a program for long-term treatment of Duchenne muscular dystrophy, experience at the University Hospital of Cleveland. *Journal of Bone and Joint Surgery, 78A*(12), 1844-1852.

Wade, D. T., & Collin, C. (1988). The Barthel ADL Index: A standard measure of physical disability? *International Disabilities Studies, 10*(2), 64-67.

Wade, D. T., & Hewer, R. L. (1987). Functional abilities after stroke: Measurement, natural history and prognosis. *Journal Neurology Neurosurgery Psychiatry, 50*, 177-182.

Walker, L. S., Van Slyke, D. A., & Newbrough, J. R. (1992). Family resources and stress: A comparison of families of children with cystic fibrosis, diabetes, and mental retardation. *Journal of Pediatric Psychology, 17*, 327-343.

Walsh, F. (1993). Conceptualization of normal family processes. In F. Walsh (Ed.), *Normal family process* (pp. 1-69). New York: Guilford.

Walsh, F. (2003). Changing families in a changing world: Reconstructing family normality. In F. Walsh (Ed.), *Normal family processes* (3 ed., pp. 3-26). New York: Guilford.

Wamboldt, M. Z., Wamboldt, F. S., Gavin, L., & Mctaggart, S. (2001). A Parent-Child Relationship Scale derived from the child and adolescent psychiatric assessment (CAPA). *Journal of the American Academy of Child & Adolescent Psychiatry, 40*(8), 945-953.

Wang, C. C., & Phinney, J. (1998). Differences in child rearing attitudes between immigrant Chinese mothers and Anglo-American mothers. *Early Development and Parenting, 7,* 181-189.

Wang, M., Jin, C., Lin, C., Wang, Y., Wu, Y., & Sun, K. (2001). [Non-invasive prenatal diagnosis of Duchenne muscular dystrophy]. *Chung-Hua i Hsueh i Chuan Hsueh Tsa Chih., 18*(2), 139-142.

Wells, K., & Whittington, D. (1993). Child and family functioning after intensive family preservation services. *Social Service Review, 67,* 55-83.

Wenniger, W. F., Hageman, W. J., & Arrindell, W. A. (1993). Cross-national validity of dimensions of family functioning: First experiences with the Dutch version of the McMaster Family Assessment Device (FAD). *Personality and Individual Differences, 14,* 769-781.

White, N., Richter, J., Koeceritz, J., & Lee, Y. A. (2002). A cross-cultural comparison of family resiliency in hemodialysis patients. *Journal of Transcultural Nursing, 13*(3), 218-227.

Wisensale, S. K. (1993). State and federal initiatives in family policy. In T. H. Brubaker (Ed.), *Family relations: Challenges for the future* (Vol. I, pp. 229-250). Newbury Park, CA: Sage.

Wu, C. C., & Huang, M. G. (1997). *A study of relation between expressed emotion and family* (RE8704-0018). Taipei, Taiwan: STIC, National Science Committee.

Wylie, C. M. (1967). Measurement and results of rehabilitation of patients with stroke. *Public Health Reports, 82,* 893-898.

Wylie, C. M., & White, B. K. (1964). A measure of disability. *Archives of Environmental Health, 8,* 834-839.

Yu, C. J. (2002). *The study of social support and self-efficacy effect to compliance with tuberculosis treatment in Taipei city.* National Yang Ming University, Taipei, Taiwan.

Appendix A

Letter of Permission I: KMU Hospital

Appendix A
Letter of Permission I: KMU Hospital

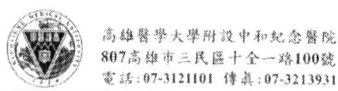

高雄醫學大學附設中和紀念醫院
807高雄市三民區十全一路100號
電話:07-3121101 傳真:07-3213931

**KAOHSIUNG MEDICAL UNIVERSITY
CHUNG-HO MEMORIAL HOSPITAL**
100 Shih-Chuan 1ˢᵗ Road, Kaohsiung 807, Taiwan
TEL: 886-7-3121101 FAX: 886-7-3213931

The Hahn School of Nursing and Science
University of San Diego
5998 Alcala Park
San Diego, Ca 92110
U.S.A.

March 27, 2003

To Whom It May Concern:

We agree that Ms. Jih-Yuan Chen to do the data collection at Kaohsiung Medical
University Chung-Ho Memorial Hospital (KMUH) for her dissertation research
project entitled: "Functioning among Families with a Child Having Duchenne
Muscular Dystrophy" during June 2003 to September 2003.

If you have any questions, please do not hesitate to contact with me.

Yours sincerely,

Shen-Long Howng, M.D., D. Med. Sc.
Superintendent
Kaohsiung Medical University
Chung-Ho Memorial Hospital

Appendix B

Letter of Permission II: TMDA

Appendix B
Letter of Permission II: TMDA

Jih-Yuan Chen
The Hahn School of Nursing and Science
University of San Diego
5998 Alcala Park
San Diego, Ca 92110
e-mail: jihc@sandiego.edu
Tel: 1-858-278-4201

I have read the information enclosed and have had it approved by the
agency IRB for the dissertation research project entitled: Functioning
among families with a child having Duchenne Muscular Dystrophy."

I agree that data collection can occur at Taiwan Muscular Dystrophy
Association during June 2003-September 2003

2003. 3. 30

Liu yung HUA   *Liu Yung HUA*
_____   _____
Signature   Date
Yung-Hua Liu
President, Taiwan Muscular Dystrophy Association
58, 3F-3, Chiou-Zuo 1st Road, San Ming District
Kaohsiung, Taiwan, ROC 80708
E-mail address: tmda168@ms22.hinet.net
Tel: 07-3801000

Appendix C

Letter of Permission: Social Worker

Appendix C
Letter of Permission III: Social Worker

Jih-Yuan Chen
The Hahn School of Nursing and Health Science
University of San Diego
5998 Alcala Park
San Diego, Ca 92110
U. S. A.

June 3, 2003

I agree to help that Ms Jih-Yuan Chen to do the research "Functioning among Families with a Child Having Duchenne Muscular Dystrophy". I will assist to counsel and support the families of children with Duchenne Muscular Dystrophy if the families have emotional risks during their processes of participation in the study.

Hui-Fang Wang   _June 3 2003_
Hui-Fang Wang   Date
Social Worker, Taiwan Muscular Dystrophy
58, 3F-3, Chiou-Zuo 1ˢᵗ Rd, San Ming District
E-mail address:tindal68@ms22.hinet.net
Tel 07-380-1000

Appendix D

Letter of Permission: Family Assessment Device

Rhode Island Hospital
A Lifespan Partner Appendix D
Letter of Permission IV: Family Assessment Device

593 Eddy Street
Providence, RI 02903

RECEIPT

TO: Jih Yuan Chen
        5998 Alcala Pk
        San Diego, CA 92110

DATE:	February 18, 2003	REFERENCE #:	CK# 1078

QUANTITY	ITEM	COST
1	McMaster Family Assessment Device	$40.00
1	McMaster Family Assessment Device – Mandarin Version	$5.00
	TOTAL AMOUNT PAID:	$45.00

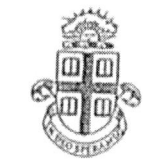

BROWN UNIVERSITY
Providence, Rhode Island 02912

Enclosed please find the FAD packet that you ordered. You have permission to duplicate the copyrighted Family Assessment Device, the manual scoring sheet and instructions, and the Family Information Form. We may contact you in the future to receive your feedback on the instrument.

Thank you for your interest and good luck in your future project.

Sincerely,

Christine E. Ryan, Ph.D.
Director, Brown University
Family Research Program
Potter 3
Rhode Island Hospital
593 Eddy Street
Providence, RI 02903

Appendix E

Letter of Permission: Duke Health Profile

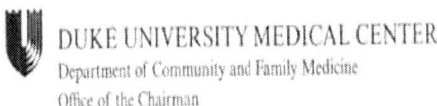

DUKE UNIVERSITY MEDICAL CENTER
Department of Community and Family Medicine
Office of the Chairman

March 28, 2003

Jih-Yuan Chen
10963 Vivaracho Way
San Diego, Ca 92124

Dear Jih-Yuan Chen,

This is to document that you have our permission to use the Duke Health Profile (DUKE) in your dissertation.

Best wishes,

George R. Parkerson, Jr.,MD, MPH
Professor of Community and Family Medicine

Appendix F

Letter of Permission: Family Hardiness Index

Appendix F
Letter of Permission VI: Family Health Index

KAMEHAMEHA SCHOOLS

Office of the Chancellor and Chief Executive Officer

April 30, 2003

Jih-Yuan Chen
10963 Vivaracho Way
San Diego, California 92124

Dear Mr. Chen:

On behalf of the developers and copyright holders of the Measure(s) that you have requested:

1) FHI: Family Hardiness Index

I would like to confirm our granting of permission to utilize this instrument for this particular investigation/study/project.

There will be no charge relating to this permission by virtue of your having required the book/CD entitled <u>Family Measures: Stress, Coping, and Resiliency</u> and have registered it accordingly.

This permission is also granted with the understanding that any revisions of these measures (e.g. language translation, etc.) will be sent to this office in its complete form to be distributed to others who may be interested in your revisions/translations.

In all cases the revisions, adaptations and the original measures, the copyright holders will remain the same as the original and also remain a property of the Kamehameha Schools and the Ke Ali'i Pauahi Foundation.

Finally, it is required that will use appropriate citation for the measure in the publication, dissertation, thesis or book. The citation that is expected in all cases will be "Published in Hamilton I. McCubbin, Ann Thompson, Marilyn McCubbin (2001) <u>Family Measures: Stress, Coping, and Resiliency</u>; Kamehameha Schools and Ke Ali'i Pauahi Foundation, Honolulu, Hawai'i."

Respectfully,

Hamilton I. McCubbin, Ph.D.
Chancellor/CEO

國 立 臺 北 護 理 學 院
中 華 民 國 臺 灣 省 臺 北 市
北 投 區 112 明 德 路 365 號
NATIONAL TAIPEI COLLEGE OF NURSING
NO. 365, MING TE ROAD, PEI TOU 112, TAIPEI
TAIWAN, REPUBLIC OF CHINA

March 10, 2003

Jih-Yuan Chen
10963 Vivaracho Way
San Diego, CA 92124
U.S.A.

Dear Miss Chen:

You have my full permission to administer my translated Chinese version of Family Hardiness Index for use in your research. Accurate credit must be given to its source where used or described in publications. I wish you success in your research and look forward to hearing the results of your investigation. Contact me any time if you have questions regarding the application of the Family Hardiness Index.

Sincerely,

Su-Chen Kuo
Associate Professor
Graduate Institute of Nurse-Midwifery
National Taipei College of Nursing
Taipei, Taiwan, R.O.C.

Appendix G

Letter of Permission--Family APGAR Scale

Date: Mon, 9 Jun 2003 17:00:53 –0400

From: Chuck Williams <Chuck.Williams@dowdenhealth.com>

To: jihc@sandiego.edu

Subject: Family APGAR

This message was written in a character set other than your own. If it is not displayed correctly, click here to open it in a new window.

Dear Ms Chen,

We are pleased to grant you permission to use the Family APGAR in your dissertation and ask only that you cite the reference thus: "Smilkstein G. The Family APGAR: A proposal for a family function test and its use by physicians. J Fam Pract 1978; 6:1231-1239."

Regards,

Chuck Williams

Charles Williams
Executive Editor
Journal of Family Practice
201-782-5708

Appendix H

Demographic Sheet

I. Family Demographic and Medical Characteristics   No: ____

Each parent should complete the instrument separately. Please mark an "v" in the box "☐" that best answers each question about your family:

Your age: _____ years
Your education level: ☐ 6 years ☐ 9 years ☐ 12 years ☐ 15 years ☐ >=15years
Your gender: ☐ male ☐ female
Your ethnicity: ☐ Taiwanese ☐ Haika ☐ Chinese ☐ aboriginal
Your relationship with DMD child: ☐ mother ☐ father
Your marital status: ☐ married ☐ separated ☐ widowed ☐ divorced
If married, quality of marital relationship: ☐ excellent ☐ good ☐ fair ☐ poor
Your employment status: ☐ employed ☐ retired ☐ homemaker
Classification of your occupation: ☐ labor ☐ technique ☐ government officer
                        ☐ professional ☐ business ☐ farmer
Your family annual income: ☐ <10,000 ☐ <15,000 ☐ <20,000 ☐ <25,000
                        ☐ =<30,000 ☐ >30,000
Satisfaction with child's medical care: ☐ yes ☐ no
Living location: ☐ rural ☐ urban ☐ municipal
Religion: ☐ Buddhism ☐ Taoist ☐ Christian ☐ Catholic ☐ none ☐ others, ____
Family structure: ☐ nuclear family ☐ extended family
Family development stage: ☐ family with preschoolers
                        ☐ family with school age children
                        ☐ family with adolescents
Number of other children: ☐1 ☐2 ☐3 ☐>3
Health condition of other children: ☐ excellent ☐ good ☐ fair ☐ poor explain:____
Family history of psychiatric disorder: ☐ yes ☐ no

Please answer the following questions about your child with Duchenne
   Muscular Dystrophy:

Child's age: _____ years
Child's education status: ☐ attend in school ☐ temporally not in school
                        ☐ permanently not in school (causes:_____)
Age of child when diagnosed with DMD _____ years
Health condition of the child: ☐ excellent ☐ good ☐ fair ☐ poor
Severity of symptom of the child: ☐ severe ☐ moderate ☐ mild

II. Child's Current Condition: Upper and Lower Extremities Functioning
   Assessment

Instructions:

Please read each statement carefully, and decide how well it describes your child's
upper extremities functioning and lower extremities functioning. You should
answer according to how you see your child's current function. Please mark an "v"
in the appropriate box "☐" about your child's upper and lower extremities
functioning.

Upper Extremities Functioning Assessment
☐ 1. Starting with arms at the sides, the child can raise and extend the arms in a
full circle until they reach above the head
☐ 2. Can raise arms above head only by flexing the elbow or using accessory
muscles
☐ 3. Can't raise hands above head, but can raise an 8-oz glass of water to the
mouth
☐ 4. Can raise hands to the mouth, but can't raise an 8-oz glass of water to the
mouth
☐ 5. Can't raise hands to the mouth, but can use hand to hold a pen or pick up
pennies from the table
☐ 6. Can't raise hands to the mouth, and has no useful function of hands

Lower Extremities Functioning Assessment:
☐ 1. Walks and climbs stairs without assistance
☐ 2. Walks and climbs stairs with aid of railing (<12 sec/4 standard steps)
☐ 3. Walks independently and climbs stairs slowly with aid of a railing (>12 sec/4
standard steps)
☐ 4. Walks independently and rises from chair unassisted but cannot climbs stairs
☐ 5. Walks independently but cannot rise from a chair or climb stairs
☐ 6. Walks independently in bilateral knee-ankle-foot orthoses
☐ 7. Walks with orthoses and assistance of one person
☐ 8. Stands in orthoses but is unable to walk even with assistance
☐ 9. Is in a wheelchair
☐ 10. Is confined to a bed

III. Child's daily activity assessment; The Barthel Index
Directions: For each activity, please mark on "v" in the appropriate box "í" about your child's daily activities.

Activity	Score
Feeding 0=unable	
5=needs help cutting, spreading butter, etc., or requires modified diet	
10=independent	_____
Bathing	
0=dependent	
5=independent (or in shower)	_____
Grooming	
0=needs to help with personal care	
5=independent face/hair/teeth/shaving (implements provided)	_____
Dressing	
0=dependent	
5=needs help but can do about half unaided	
10=independent (including buttons, zips, laces, etc.)	_____
Bowels	
0=incontinent (or needs to be given enemas)	
5=occasional accident	
10=continent	_____
Bladder	
0=incontinent, or catheterized and unable to manage alone	
5=occasional accident	
10=continent	_____
Toilet Use	
0=dependent	
5=needs some help, but can do something alone	
10=independent (on and off, dressing, wiping)	_____
Transfers (Bed to chair and back)	
0=unable, no sitting balance	
5=major help (one or two people, physical), can sit	
10=minor help (verbal or physical)	
15=independent	_____
Mobility (on level surfaces)	
0=immobile or < 50 yards	
5=wheelchair independent, including corners, > 50 yards	
10=walks with help of one person (verbal or physical) > 50 yards	
15=independent (but may use any aid; for example, stick) > 50 yards	_____
Stairs	
0=unable	
5=needs help (verbal, physical, carrying aid)	
10=independent	_____
Total (0-100):	_____

Appendix I
Duke Health Profile (The DUKE)

Instructions: Here are some questions about your health and feelings. Please read each question carefully and check (v) your best answer. You should answer the questions in your own way. There are no right or wrong answers. (Please ignore the small scoring numbers next each blank.)

	Yes, describes me exactly	Somewhat describe me	No, doesn't describe me at all
1. I like who I am	2	1	0
2. I am not an easy person to get along with	0	1	2
3. I am basically a healthy person	2	1	0
4. I give up too easily	0	1	2
5. I have difficulty concentrating	0	1	2
6. I am happy with my family relationships	2	1	0
7. I am comfortable being around people	2	1	0

Today would you have any physical trouble or difficulty?

	None	Some	A Lot
8. Walking up a flight of stairs	2	1	0
9. Running the length of a football field	2	1	0

During the past week: How much trouble have you had with

	None	Some	A Lot
10. Sleeping	2	1	0
11. Hurting or aching in any part of your body	2	1	0
12. Getting tired easily	2	1	0
13. Feeling depressed or sad	2	1	0
14. Nervousness	2	1	0

During the past week: How often did you

	None	Some	A Lot
15. Socialize with other people (talk or visit with friends or relatives)	0	1	2
16. Take part in social, religious, or recreation activities (meetings, church, movies, sports, parties)	0	1	2

During the past week: How often did you

	None	1-4 Days	5-7 Days
17. Stay in your home, a nursing home, or hospital because of sickness, injury, or other health problem	2	1	0

Appendix J

Family APGAR Scale

The following questions have been designed to help us better understand you and your family. You should feel free to ask questions about any item in the questionnaire. Please try to answer all questions

Family is the individual(s) with whom you usually live. If you live alone, consider family as those with whom you now have the strongest emotional ties.

For each question, check only one box

	Almost always	Some of the time	Never
I am satisfied that I can turn to my family for help when something is troubling me	2 ☐	1 ☐	0 ☐
I am satisfied with the way my family talks over things with me and shares problems with me	2 ☐	1 ☐	0 ☐
I am satisfied that my family accepts and supports my wishes to take on new activities or directions	2 ☐	1 ☐	0 ☐
I am satisfied with the way my family expresses affection and responds to my emotion, such as anger, sorrow, or love	2 ☐	1 ☐	0 ☐
I am satisfied with the way my family and I share time together	2 ☐	1 ☐	0 ☐

Appendix K

Family Hardiness Index

Directions:

Please read each statement below and decide to what degree each describes your family. Is the statement false (0), mostly false (1), mostly true (2), or true (3) about your family? Circle a number 0 to 3 to match your feelings about each statement. Please respond to each and every statement.

In our family......	False	Mostly False	Mostly True	True	
1. Trouble results from mistakes we make	0	1	2	3	®
2. It is not wise to plan ahead and hope because things do not turn out anyway	0	1	2	3	®
3. Our work and effort are not appreciated no matter how hard we try and work	0	1	2	3	®
4. In the long run, the bad things that happen to us are balanced by the good things that happen	0	1	2	3	
5. We have a sense of being strong even when we face big problems	0	1	2	3	
6. Many times I feel I can trust that even in difficult times things will work out	0	1	2	3	
7. While we don't always agree, we can count on each other to stand by us in times of need	0	1	2	3	
8. We do not feel we can survive if another problem hits us	0	1	2	3	®
9. We believe that things will work out for the better if we work together as a family	0	1	2	3	
10. Life seems dull and meaningless	0	1	2	3	®
11. We strive together and help each other no matter what	0	1	2	3	
12. When our family plans activities we try new and exciting things	0	1	2	3	
13. We listen to each others' problems, hurts and fears	0	1	2	3	
14. We tend to do the same things over and over...it's boring	0	1	2	3	®
15. We seem to encourage each other to try new things and experiences	0	1	2	3	
16. It is better to stay at home than go out and do things with others	0	1	2	3	®
17. Being active and learning new things are encouraged	0	1	2	3	
18. We work together to solve problems	0	1	2	3	
19. Most of the unhappy things that happen are due to bad luck	0	1	2	3	®
20. We realize our lives are controlled by accidents and luck	0	1	2	3	®

The ® symbol is for computer use only   Total_____

Appendix L

Family Assessment Device

Appendix L

FAMILY ASSESSMENT DEVICE
Brown University/Rhode Island Hospital Family Research Program

INSTRUCTIONS:

This booklet contains a number of statements about families. Please read each statement carefully, and decide how well it describes your own family. You should answer according to how you see your family.

For each statement there are four (4) possible responses:

Strongly Agree (SA)	Check SA if you feel that the statement describes your family very accurately.
Agree (A)	Check A if you feel that the statement describes your family for the most part.
Disagree (D)	Check D if you feel that the statement does not describe your family for the most part.
Strongly Disagree (SD)	Check SD if you feel that the statement does not describe you family at all.

These four responses will appear below each statement like this:

41. We are not satisfied with anything short of perfection.

_____ SA _____ A _____ D _____ SD   _____

The answer spaces for statement 41 would look like this. For each statement in the booklet, there is an answer space below. Do not pay attention to the blanks at the far right-hand side of each space. They are for office use only.

Try not to spend too much time thinking about each statement, but respond as quickly and as honestly as you can. If you have trouble with one, answer with your first reaction. Please be sure to answer every statement and mark all your answers in the space provided below each statement.

FAMILY ASSESSMENT DEVICE
Brown University/Rhode Island Hospital Family Research Program

ID _____

Page 1

1. Planning family activities is difficult because we misunderstand each other.

_____ SA _____ A _____ D _____ SD

_____

2. We resolve most everyday problems around the house.

_____ SA _____ A _____ D _____ SD

_____

3. When someone is upset the others know why.

_____ SA _____ A _____ D _____ SD

_____

4. When you ask someone to do something, you have to check that they did it.

_____ SA _____ A _____ D _____ SD

_____

5. If someone is in trouble, the others become too involved.

_____ SA _____ A _____ D _____ SD

_____

6. In times of crisis we can turn to each other for support.

_____ SA _____ A _____ D _____ SD

_____

7. We don't know what to do when an emergency comes up.

_____ SA _____ A _____ D _____ SD

_____

8. We sometimes run out of things that we need.

_____ SA _____ A _____ D _____ SD

_____

9. We are reluctant to show our affection for each other.

_____ SA _____ A _____ D _____ SD

_____

10. We make sure members meet their family responsibilities.

_____ SA _____ A _____ D _____ SD

_____

11. We cannot talk to each other about the sadness we feel.

_____ SA _____ A _____ D _____ SD

_____

12. We usually act on our decisions regarding problems.

_____SA _____A _____D _____SD

13. You only get the interest of others when something is important to them.

_____SA _____A _____D _____SD

14. You can't tell how a person is feeling from what they are saying.

_____SA _____A _____D _____SD

15. Family tasks don't get spread around enough.

_____SA _____A _____D _____SD

16. Individuals are accepted for what they are.

_____SA _____A _____D _____SD

17. You can easily get away with breaking the rules.

_____SA _____A _____D _____SD

18. People come right out and say things instead of hinting at them.

_____SA _____A _____D _____SD

19. Some of us just don't respond emotionally.

_____SA _____A _____D _____SD

20. We know what to do in an emergency.

_____SA _____A _____D _____SD

21. We avoid discussing our fears and concerns.

_____SA _____A _____D _____SD

22. It is difficult to talk to each other about tender feelings.

_____SA _____A _____D _____SD

23. We have trouble meeting our bills.

_____SA   _____A   _____D   _____SD   _____

24. After our family tries to solve a problem, we usually discuss whether it worked or not.

_____SA   _____A   _____D   _____SD   _____

25. We are too self-centered.

_____SA   _____A   _____D   _____SD   _____

26. We can express feelings to each other.

_____SA   _____A   _____D   _____SD   _____

27. We have no clear expectations about toilet habits.

_____SA   _____A   _____D   _____SD   _____

28. We do not show our love for each other.

_____SA   _____A   _____D   _____SD   _____

29. We talk to people directly rather than through go-betweens.

_____SA   _____A   _____D   _____SD   _____

30. Each of us has particular duties and responsibilities.

_____SA   _____A   _____D   _____SD   _____

31. There are lots of bad feelings in the family.

_____SA   _____A   _____D   _____SD   _____

32. We have rules about hitting people.

_____SA   _____A   _____D   _____SD   _____

33. We get involved with each other only when something interest us.

_____SA   _____A   _____D   _____SD   _____

34. There's little time to explore personal interests.

_____SA   _____A   _____D   _____SD   _____

35. We often don't say what we mean.

_____SA   _____A   _____D   _____SD   _____

36. We feel accepted for what we are.

_____SA   _____A   _____D   _____SD   _____

37. We show interest in each other when we can get something out of it personally.

_____SA   _____A   _____D   _____SD   _____

38. We resolve most emotional upsets that come up.

_____SA   _____A   _____D   _____SD   _____

39. Tenderness takes second place to other things in our family.

_____SA   _____A   _____D   _____SD   _____

40. We discuss who is to do household jobs.

_____SA   _____A   _____D   _____SD   _____

41. Making decisions is a problem for our family.

_____SA   _____A   _____D   _____SD   _____

42. Our family shows interest in each other only when they can get something out of it.

_____SA   _____A   _____D   _____SD   _____

43. We are frank with each other.

_____SA   _____A   _____D   _____SD   _____

44. We don't hold to any rules or standards.

_____SA   _____A   _____D   _____SD   _____

45. If people are asked to do something, they need reminding.

_____SA _____A _____D _____SD   _____

46. We are able to make decisions about how to solve problems.

_____SA _____A _____D _____SD   _____

47. If the rules are broken, we don't know what to expect.

_____SA _____A _____D _____SD   _____

48. Anything goes in our family.

_____SA _____A _____D _____SD   _____

49. We express tenderness.

_____SA _____A _____D _____SD   _____

50. We confront problems involving feelings.

_____SA _____A _____D _____SD   _____

51. We don't get along well together.

_____SA _____A _____D _____SD   _____

52. We don't talk to each other when we are angry.

_____SA _____A _____D _____SD   _____

53. We are generally dissatisfied with the family duties assigned to us.

_____SA _____A _____D _____SD   _____

54. Even though we mean well, we intrude too much into each others lives.

_____SA _____A _____D _____SD   _____

55. There are rules about dangerous situations.

_____SA _____A _____D _____SD   _____

FAMILY ASSESSMENT DEVICE
Brown University/Rhode Island Hospital Family Research Program

ID _____ _____
Page 6

56. We confide in each other.

_____ SA   _____ A   _____ D   _____ SD   _____

57. We cry openly.

_____ SA   _____ A   _____ D   _____ SD   _____

58. We don't have reasonable transport.

_____ SA   _____ A   _____ D   _____ SD   _____

59. When we don't like what someone has done, we tell them.

_____ SA   _____ A   _____ D   _____ SD   _____

60. We try to think of different ways to solve problems.

_____ SA   _____ A   _____ D   _____ SD   _____

Appendix M
Information Sheet for the Subjects

Researcher
    Jih-Yuan Chen, PhD. Candidate, MSN, RN.
    Doctoral Student
    Hahn School of Nursing and Health Science
    University of San Diego
    (858) 278-4201
    jihc@sandiego.edu
Faculty Advisor
    Susan L. Instone, DNSc, RN, CPNP
    Hahn School of Nursing and Health Science
    University of San Diego
    5998 Alcala Park
    San Diego, Ca 92110
    (619) 260-4549
    sinstone@sandiego.edu

Purpose and Explanation
Jih-Yuan Chen, a doctoral candidate at the University of San Diego, is doing a research study to learn more about how Taiwanese families with a child having Duchenne muscular dystrophy (DMD) function. As a parent of a child with DMD, you are being asked to participate. Ms. Chen will collect and analyze the data in this study. Dr. Instone serves as the faculty advisor. Ms. Chen may consult with Dr. Instone and the other members of her dissertation committee from the University of San Diego regarding data analysis.

Procedures
If you agree to participate in the study, the following will occur
1. You will be called by Ms. Chen and asked to participate voluntarily in the study.
2. You will be given a chance to ask questions about this research study before you are asked to sign the consent form.
3. You will be sent the questionnaires by mail. These include the Demographic Sheet (including family and medical characteristics, child's upper and lower extremities functioning, and child's daily activity), the Duke Health Profile-17 items, Family APGAR Scale-5 items, Family Hardiness Index-20 items, and Family Assessment Device-60 items. It will take about one hour to complete these questionnaires.
4. Please answer the questions within 2 weeks at a convenient time. The researcher will be available by phone or face to face if you need help answering the questions. If for any reason you do not
wish to answer the question, you may stop at any time.
5. Your participation is voluntary and may be terminated at any time for any reason.
6. Any information shared with Ms Chen will not be shared with any others. All information will be confidential.

Risks/Discomforts
    You have been informed that participation in this study may involve few emotional risks. If counseling or support is needed, you may call social worker Miss Hui-Fong Wang 07-380-1000 at the Taiwan Muscular Dystrophy Association.

Benefits
    You will receive no benefit from participating in this study. Ms Chen may achieve a better understanding of what factors influence family functioning in families with a child having a DMD. In addition, the study may contribute knowledge to the development of intervention that will help to promote better functioning.

Appendix N

Consent Form

Project: Functioning Among Taiwanese Families with a Child Having Duchenne
     Muscular Dystrophy
Researcher: Jih-Yuan Chen, RN, MSN
Ms. Chen is an Associate Professor at the College of Nursing of Kaohsiung Medical
University, and a doctoral student conducting research for a dissertation at the University of
San Diego, USA.

The purpose of the study is to investigate the factors associated with functioning among
families with a child having Duchenne Muscular Dystrophy. If you agree to be in the study,
you will complete four written questionnaires: Family Hardiness Index (FHI), Family
APGAR, Family Assessment Device (FAD), Duke Health Profile (Duke), and Demographic
sheet. These questionnaires are expected to take one hour to complete.

You will be free to telephone the researcher: Ms. Jih-Yuan Chen 07-3233778 (Taiwan) or
002-1-858-278-4201 (USA), and Dr. Susan Instone 002-1-619-260-4549 (USA) with any
questions you may have. Your name will not appear on any of these questionnaires.
Furthermore, all information provided in the questionnaires will be treated in a confidential
manner. All data will be locked in a file cabinet with access only by the investigator. All data
will be destroyed in five years.

This study will not provide any direct benefits to you, but the results of the study may
influence the quality of life of others families in the future. You have been informed that
participation in this study may involve few emotional risks. If counseling or support is
needed, you may call social worker Miss Hui-Fong Wang 07-380-1000 at the Taiwan
Muscular Dystrophy Association. You may decide to withdraw at any time, and your child's
medical care will not be affected in any way if you decide to withdraw.

Completing the questionnaires will take about one hour. I have been given the opportunity to
ask whatever questions I desire.

_____   _____

Signature of Participant   Date

_____

Location

_____   _____

Signature of Researcher   Date

Appendix O

Appendix O
Human Subjects Approval from the University of San Diego

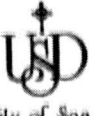

University of San Diego

Institutional Review Board

Project Action Summary

Action Date: 6/4/03   *Note: Approval expires one year after this date.*

Type: __New Full Review _X_New Expedited Review ___Continuation Review ___Exempt Review
         ____Modification

Action: _X__Approved   ____Approved Pending Modification   ___Not Approved

   2003-06-104
       Ms. Jih-Yuan Chen Doc Nurs
       Dr. Susan Instone Fac Nurs
       "Functioning Among Taiwanese Families With a Child Having Duchenne Muscular Distrophy."

   *Note: We send IRB correspondence regarding student research to the faculty advisor, who bears
           the ultimate responsibility for the conduct of the research. We request that the faculty advisor
           share this correspondence with the student researcher.*

Modifications Required or Reasons for Non-Approval

Approved.

The next deadline for submitting project proposals to the Provost's Office for full review is _____. You
may submit a project proposal for expedited review at any time.

Dr. Donald J. McGraw
Administrator, Institutional Review Board
mcgraw@sandiego.edu

參與研究對象的說明指引

研究者

陳季員，博士候選人，理學碩士，護理師

Hahn 護理健康學院博士班學生，美國聖地亞哥大學

電話：002-1-858-278-4201, 07-3233778

E-mail：jihc@sandiego.edu

指導教授：Susan L. Instone 博士

美國聖地亞哥大學，Hahn 護理健康學院

5998 Alcala Park, San Diego CA92124

電話：002-1-619-260-4549

E-mail：sinstone@sandiego.edu

目的和解釋

陳季員，係美國聖地亞哥大學博士候選人，正從事研究以得知有關台灣杜顯型肌肉萎縮兒童家庭的功能，身為肌肉萎縮兒童的父母將被邀請參與此研究，陳女士將在本研究中收集資料並分析資料，Instone 博士則擔任指導教授，陳女士將諮詢 Instone 博士和聖地亞哥大學 Hahn 護理健康學院博士論文委員會的其他委員。

方法

如果您同意參與此研究，將依下列步驟進行：

1. 陳女士將以電話聯繫，徵求您的同意，自願參與。
2. 您簽同意書之前，有任何疑問將給以機會詢問。
3. 您接到郵寄的問卷，這份問卷包含人口學調查表，杜氏健康評估表，家庭關懷度指數量表，家庭耐力量表，和家庭功能量表。
4. 請盡可能在二星期內，您方便的時間內填寫問卷表並寄回，填寫問卷約需花費一個小時，若基於某些原因您不想回答問題，您可以隨時終止。
5. 您的參與是自願性的，也可以隨時終止。
6. 任何和陳女士分享的資料並不會讓別人得知，所有資料是保密的且反鎖，資料在五年內並定銷毀。

危機/不適

您參與此研究也許會有些微的情緒伏動，如果有需要諮詢或支持，您可以電話聯繫王慧芳小姐 07-3800566。

利益

您參與此研究將不會收到任何利益，但有您的協助，陳女士可以獲得更佳的了解影響杜顯型肌肉萎縮兒童家庭功能的因素，此外，這研究對發展促進更佳功能的知識會有貢獻。

同意書

計畫名稱：台灣杜顯型肌肉萎縮兒童家庭的功能

研究者：陳季員，理學碩士，護理師

陳女士係高雄醫學大學護理學院副教授，同時也是美國聖地亞哥大學，Hahn 護理健康學院博士班學生，正在進行博士論文研究。

這研究的目的是發現杜顯型肌肉萎縮兒童家庭功能的相關因素，如果您同意參與此研究，您將填寫五份問卷表：人口學調查表，杜氏健康評估表，家庭關懷度指數量表，家庭耐力量表，和家庭功能量表。填寫問卷約需花費一個小時。

如果您有任何問題可以隨時打電話給研究者陳季員女士 07-3233778，或 Susan Instone 博士 002-1-619-260-4549 (美國)。您的名字將不會出現在任何問卷表上，而且所有問卷表上的信息將是保密狀態，所有資料將鎖在資料櫃內，只有研究者可以接近，所有資料將在五年內銷毀。

這研究對您不會提供任何直接的利益，但研究結果可能影響將來其他家庭的生活品質，在這研究不會因為您的參與而對您有健康上的危害，任何時間您可以決定退出，如您決定退出也將不會影響您的醫療照護。

將需花一小時完成問卷，我也曾有機會詢問我想問的問題。

_____   _____
參與者簽名   日期

_____
地點

_____   _____
研究者簽名   日期

_____   _____
見證者   日期

杜氏(DUKE)健康評估量表

說明：下列為許多有關您的健康和感覺的問題。

　　　請仔細讀每一問題並勾選(ˇ)最適合您的答案。您應該以您自己的情形來回答這些問題，答案並沒有對或錯。

	是的，這正描述我的情形	多少有點描述我的情形	不，這一點也不描述我的情形
1. 我喜歡我這個樣子	( )	( )	( )
2. 我覺得我不是一個容易相處的人	( )	( )	( )
3. 基本上，我是一個健康的人	( )	( )	( )
4. 我太容易放棄	( )	( )	( )
5. 我難以專心	( )	( )	( )
6. 我非常滿意我的家庭關係	( )	( )	( )
7. 我覺得與人相處會自在	( )	( )	( )

今天，您從事下列活動，您是否會有任何生理上的不適或困難：

	完全沒有	有一些	很大
8. 爬上一層樓的樓梯	( )	( )	( )
9. 跑 100 公尺	( )	( )	( )

在過去的一星期中，對於下列情況，您曾有過多少困擾：

	完全沒有	有一些	很大
10. 睡眠	( )	( )	( )
11. 您身體任何部位的疼痛	( )	( )	( )
12. 容易變得疲倦	( )	( )	( )
13. 感到沮喪或悲傷	( )	( )	( )
14. 感到精神緊張	( )	( )	( )

在過去的一星期中：您多常會做下列的事？

	完全不曾	有時	經常
15. 其他人交往〔講話、拜訪朋友或親戚〕	( )	( )	( )
16. 參與社交、宗教或娛樂活動〔集會、教堂、電影、運動、聚會〕	( )	( )	( )

在過去的一星期中：您多常會：

	完全不曾	1-4 天	5-7 天
17. 因為生病、受傷或其他健康問題，待在家裡、護理之家或是醫院	( )	( )	( )

好，接下來看看您家人的關懷支持狀況！

家庭關懷度指數量表 (Family APGAR)

說明：

下列的問題是幫助我們更了解您和您的家庭，您可以自由地並試著回答所有的每一項目；家人是指和您住在一起的所有人，若您現在是獨處，則考慮家人是指和您現在有強烈的情感聯結的人，將最適合您的答案，請在每一題的括號( )內打勾 "✓"。

	總是 如此	有時 如此	很少 如此
1. 當您有麻煩或煩惱時，你可以從家庭得到幫助。	( )	( )	( )
2. 您很滿意家人和您討論事情及分擔問題的方式	( )	( )	( )
3. 當您想要做一種新的事情時，家庭會給您滿意的接受和支持。	( )	( )	( )
4. 您很滿意家人對您的情緒（喜、怒、哀、樂）表示關心和愛護的方式。	( )	( )	( )
5. 您和家人可以共度愉快的時光。	( )	( )	( )

很好，我們再評估您的家庭耐力支持狀況：

家庭耐力量表 (Family Hardiness Index)

說明：此部分是要瞭解您對家庭的感覺，針對每一題描述您家庭狀況，**請圈選最符合您感覺的數字**，０是完全錯誤的，１是大部分錯誤的，２是大部分正確的，３是完全正確的。

在我們家裡……

	完全錯誤的	大部分錯誤的	大部分正確的	完全正確的
1.麻煩是因為我們所犯的錯誤	0	1	2	3
2.事先計畫和預期是不明智的，因為不管怎樣事情總不會如預期的	0	1	2	3
3.不管我們如何努力和工作，我們的工作和辛勞都是不被賞識的	0	1	2	3
4.到頭來，發生在我們身上的不好事情，會被所發生的好事情所補償	0	1	2	3
5.即使面對重大的問題，我們仍有堅強的感覺	0	1	2	3
6.很多時候，我覺得我可以相信即使在困難的時刻，事情終會解決的	0	1	2	3
7.雖然我們常有意見不合的時候，但在需要幫助的時刻，我們可以相信彼此是互相支持的	0	1	2	3
8.假如有另外的問題再發生，我們不認為我們能應付得了	0	1	2	3
9.我們相信假如一家人同心協力，事情會有更好的解決	0	1	2	3
10.生活似乎是無聊和無意義的	0	1	2	3
11.不論發生任何事，我們一起奮鬥和互相幫忙	0	1	2	3
12.當我們計畫家庭活動時，我們會嘗試新鮮的、令人興奮的事情	0	1	2	3
13.我們聆聽、感受彼此的問題、痛苦和害怕	0	1	2	3
14.我們一再做相同的事情，這真是無聊	0	1	2	3
15.我們似乎是鼓勵彼此去嘗試新的事情和經驗	0	1	2	3
16.留在家裡比外出與他人一起做事更好	0	1	2	3
17.主動學習新的事情是受到鼓勵的	0	1	2	3

在我們家裡……	完全錯誤的	大部分錯誤的	大部分正確的	完全正確的
18.我們一起設法解決問題	0	1	2	3
19.大多數不愉快事情之所以會發生，是由於運氣不好	0	1	2	3
20.我們瞭解我們的生活是被不可預料的事情和運氣所控制的	0	1	2	3

再接再厲，來評估您家庭的功能!

家庭評估工具 (Family Assessment Device)：家庭功能

　　說明：此部分包含許多有關家庭的描述，針對每一題描述您家庭狀況，根據您所看到自己的家庭，請仔細讀並決定最符合您自己家庭的描述，請圈上最適合您感覺家庭實際情況的號碼：1 非常同意--是指感覺完全正確的描述您的家庭，

2 同意--是指感覺大部分正確的描述您的家庭 3 不同意--是指感覺大部分不是描述您的家庭， 4 絕對不同意--是指感覺完全不是描述您的家庭。

	非常同意	同意	不同意	絕對不同意
1. 計劃全家性的活動異常困難，原因在於我們常彼此誤會	1	2	3	4
2. 我們都能解決家中大部分的日常問題	1	2	3	4
3. 當一個家人感到不開心的時候，其他家人會曉得個中原因	1	2	3	4
4. 當你吩咐家中某人做些事時，你一要去查看他是否有做	1	2	3	4
5. 當一個家人遇有困難，其他家人常會過份關心	1	2	3	4
6. 當危機來到時，我們可從家人獲得支持	1	2	3	4
7. 在危急關頭，我們往往不知如何應對	1	2	3	4
8. 家中常缺乏需要的物品	1	2	3	4
9. 我們不願向家人表達愛心與關心	1	2	3	4
10. 我們堅持要家中各人肩負對家庭的責任	1	2	3	4
11. 當我感到憂傷時，也不會向家人傾訴	1	2	3	4
12. 當我們對問題作出對策時，我們通常會實行此項對策	1	2	3	4
13. 其他家人對於我的事情都不感興趣，除非那件事對他們也有重要性	1	2	3	4
14. 我們不能從一個家人的說話去分辨他的感受	1	2	3	4
15. 家務的分配並不平均	1	2	3	4
16. 每個人是毫無條件地被接納	1	2	3	4
17. 不守規矩，也不一定受處分	1	2	3	4
18. 我們有話便直說，不會含蓄或半吞半吐	1	2	3	4
19. 我們有些人從不表露感情	1	2	3	4
20. 我們曉得如何應付危急關頭	1	2	3	4
21. 我們避開談論各人所恐懼及擔心的事	1	2	3	4
22. 談論自己溫柔一面的感受是尷尬的事	1	2	3	4
23. 我們不夠錢付賬單	1	2	3	4
24. 當我們一家嘗試解決一些問題之後，我們往往會討論這方法是否有效	1	2	3	4
25. 我們太自我中心	1	2	3	4

請圈上最符合您家庭實際情況的號碼	非常同意	同意	不同意	絕對不同意
26. 我們可彼此吐露真情	1	2	3	4
27. 對於使用洗手間的習慣，我們從不說清楚對於彼此的期望	1	2	3	4
28. 我們從不表達對大家的期望與愛	1	2	3	4
29. 我們可直接溝通，不需要任何的「中間人」	1	2	3	4
30. 各人都有特別的責任與任	1	2	3	4
31. 我們對家人有許多積怨	1	2	3	4
32. 對於動手打人，我們有清楚的規矩	1	2	3	4
33. 我們不會關心其他人的事，除非我們對那件事也感興趣	1	2	3	4
34. 我們沒有時間探索個人的興趣	1	2	3	4
35. 我們不會說真心話	1	2	3	4
36. 我們感覺到被接納	1	2	3	4
37. 我們不會對其他家人的事感興趣，除非我們能從中取到個人利益	1	2	3	4
38. 我們多能解決情緒上的波動	1	2	3	4
39. 我們不太重視彼此溫和相對	1	2	3	4
40. 我們一起商討家務的分配	1	2	3	4
41. 對我們一家來說，做決定是很困難的事	1	2	3	4
42. 除非我們可從中取利，否則不會對其他家人感興趣	1	2	3	4
43. 我們可坦誠相對	1	2	3	4
44. 我們並不持守任何規則或標準	1	2	3	4
45. 當你吩咐一個家人做點事，你需提醒他	1	2	3	4
46. 我們面對問題，往往能做出決定如何去解決	1	2	3	4
47. 如果家中的規矩不被遵守，我們便不知期望什麼了	1	2	3	4
48. 什麼事都許可的	1	2	3	4
49. 我們可表達溫柔一面的感受	1	2	3	4
50. 當遇到一些問題，是涉及個人的感受時，我們也可以正面面對	1	2	3	4
51. 我們相處並不融洽	1	2	3	4
52. 當我們感到憤怒之時，便不睬其他人	1	2	3	4

請圈上最符合您家庭實際情況的號碼

	非常同意	同意	不同意	絕對不同意
53. 我們並不滿意家務與責任的分配	1	2	3	4
54. 雖然我們是出於好意，卻過分闖進其他家人的生活範圍	1	2	3	4
55. 對於危險的情況，我們都有規則	1	2	3	4
56. 我們彼此信任	1	2	3	4
57. 我們可在家人面前哭	1	2	3	4
58. 我們缺乏合理的交通工具	1	2	3	4
59. 如果我們不滿某家人之所爲，便會告訴他	1	2	3	4
60. 我們嘗試思想不同的方法來解決問題	1	2	3	4

最後請協助評估您孩子的當前的狀況!

I.上肢功能評估 (請圈上最符合您孩子的當前實際情況的號碼)
1. 手臂能輕易自身旁兩側外展舉起超過頭的高度。
2. 需運用輔具肌肉及彎曲手肘才能將手舉高至頭頂。
3. 不能將手舉高超過頭頂，但能拿起一杯 250c.c.的水到口(必要時可用兩手)。
4. 能舉起手到口，但不能拿起一杯 250c.c.的水到口。
5. 不能舉起手到口，但手能握筆或自桌上撿起銅板。
6. 不能舉起手到口，手亦無有用的功能。

II.下肢功能評估(請圈上最符合您孩子的當前實際情況的號碼)
1. 走路和爬樓梯時不需協助。
2. 走路和爬樓梯時需扶著扶手(小於 12 秒/4 階樓梯)。
3. 走路和爬樓梯時需扶著扶手(大於 12 秒/4 階樓梯)。
4. 可獨自走路及從椅子上站起來，但不能爬樓梯。
5. 可獨自走路，但不能獨自從椅子上站起來或爬樓梯。
6. 走路需協助或需借助於長鐵鞋。
7. 走路需著長鐵鞋且需協助以保持平衡。
8. 能著長鐵鞋站立，但即使受助亦不能走路。
9. 坐輪椅。
0. 躺在床上。

III. 日常生活依賴狀況

巴氏日常生活量表 (Barthel Index)

說明：請在各項日常活動的 " □ " 內，圈上 "v" 最符合您孩子的當前實際情況：

進食
　　□：自己在合理的時間內 (約 10 秒吃一口) 可用筷子取食眼前的食物，若
　　　　需使用進食輔具，應會自行穿脫。
　　□：需別人幫忙穿脫進食輔具，或只會用湯匙進食。
　　□：無法自行取食，或耗費的時間過長。
洗澡
　　□：可以獨立完成洗澡。
　　□：需要幫忙洗澡。
個人衛生
　　□：可以獨立完成洗臉、洗手、刷牙、梳頭法及刮鬍子。
　　□：需要別人幫忙完成洗臉、洗手、刷牙、梳頭法及刮鬍子的工作。
穿脫衣服
　　□：可以自行穿脫衣服、鞋子及輔具。
　　□：在別人幫忙下，可自行完成一半以上的動作。
　　□：需要別人幫忙。
大便控制
　　□：大便不會失禁，並自行使用塞劑。
　　□：偶爾會大便失禁 (每週不超過一次)，或使用塞劑時需別人幫忙。
　　□：需別人處理。
小便控制
　　□：日夜皆不會尿失禁。或可自行使用並清理尿套。
　　□：偶爾會尿失禁 (每週不超過一次)，或尿急 (無法等待便盆或無法及
　　　　時趕到廁所)，或需別人幫忙處理尿套。
　　□：需別人處理。
如廁
　　□：可自行進出廁所，不會弄髒衣服，並能穿好衣服使用便盆，可自行清
　　　　理便盆。
　　□：需幫忙保持姿勢的平衡，整理衣物或使用衛生紙使用便盆，可自行取
　　　　放便盆但需賴他人清理。
　　□：需賴別人處理上廁所的問題。

輪椅與床位之間的移位
　　□：可獨立完成，包括輪椅的煞車及移開腳踏板。
　　□：需要稍微協助 (例如予以輕扶以保持平衡) 或口頭指導。
　　□：可自行從床上坐起來，但移位時仍需別人幫忙。
　　□：需別人幫忙方可坐起來或需兩人幫忙方可移位。

行走平地上
　　□：使用或不使用輔具皆可獨立行走 50 公尺以上，穿長鐵支架者，
　　　　可自行適時的固定及鬆脫。
　　□：需要稍微的扶持或口頭指導方可行走 50 公尺以上。
　　□：雖無法行走，但可獨立操縱輪椅 (包括轉彎、進門及接近桌子、
　　　　床沿) 並可推行輪椅 50 公尺以上。
　　□：需別人幫忙推輪椅。
上下樓梯
　　□：可自行走上下樓梯 (允許抓扶手、用枴杖)。
　　□：需稍微幫忙或口頭指導而能上下樓梯。
　　□：無法上下樓梯。

再請撥冗填寫基本的資料

人口學基本的資料

I.　　人口學的和醫學的資料

說明：請每位父母務必各自填答，針對您及家庭的每一問題，請在最符合的 " □ "
　　　內打 " ∨ "

您的年齡: _____ 歲
您的教育程度: □6 年 □9 年 □12 年 □15 年 □>=15 年
您的性別: □男 □女
您的祖籍: □台灣省籍 □客家籍 □大陸省籍 □原著民
您與孩子的關係: □父子 □母子
您的婚姻狀況: □已婚 □分居 □鰥寡 □離婚
已婚的您，婚姻關係: □非常好 □很好 □尚好 □不好
您的就業狀況: □就業 □退休 □家庭主婦
您的職業別: □勞工 □技術人員 □行政事務、公務人員 □專門職業人員
　　　　□從商 □務農
您家庭的月收入: □<=30,000 □<=45,000 □<=60,000 □<=75,000
　　　　　　　　□<=90,000 □<=105,000 □<=120,000 □<135,000
　　　　　　　　□<=150,000 □>150,000
您滿意孩子的醫療照顧: □是 □否
您住家位於: □鄉村 □城鎮 □院轄市
您的宗教信仰: □佛教 □道教 □基督教 □天主教 □其他_____
您的家庭結構: □核心家庭 □擴展家庭
您的家庭發展階段: □有學齡前期兒童家庭 □有學齡兒童家庭 □有青少年家庭
家庭精神疾病史: □有 □無

請回答下列有關杜顯型肌萎縮孩子的問題
您孩子的年齡: _____ 歲
您孩子的教育狀況: □就學 □暫未就學 □不再就學 (未就學原因_____)
您孩子被診斷為杜顯型肌萎縮是幾歲？_____ 歲
您孩子的健康狀況: □非常好 □很好 □尚好 □不好(請說明_____)
您孩子的病症嚴重度: □重度嚴重 □中度嚴重 □輕度嚴重
您孩子的手足之健康狀況: □非常好 □很好 □尚好 □不好(請說明_____)

感謝您完成整份的問卷
祝福闔家健康快樂

Printed in the United Kingdom by
Lightning Source UK Ltd., Milton Keynes
137140UK00001B/296/P